PRAISE FOR *RESTORING OUR GIRLS*

"*Restoring Our Girls* empowers parents by offering them a blueprint for engaging in the real conversation our girls so desperately need right now. With compassion and empathy, Adams guides parents to focus on what really matters: listening, understanding, and supporting our daughters. In the process, Adams also offers critical insights that enable parents to gain a deeper understanding of themselves. This is a game-changing book for modern parents who want their daughters to thrive in adolescence and beyond."

—**Jennifer Breheny Wallace**, author of the *New York Times* bestselling book *Never Enough: When Achievement Culture Becomes Toxic—And What We Can Do About It*

"By masterfully equipping parents with skills to engage in conscious communication with their teen daughters, this critically essential book is aimed to help both navigate and thrive through the storms of adolescence in a way that not only keeps them connected, but allows the children to emerge as empowered adults. A book I wish my parents had during my teen years, this is an urgent and priceless read."

—**Dr. Shefali**, clinical psychologist and *NYT* bestselling author

"If you once marveled at the spirit and personality of your little girl but find yourself baffled lately at where that vibrant person has gone, read this book. Cathy tackles the systemic, political, and cultural issues that complicate girlhood today, in the process giving parents the language to confidently and convincingly talk with their daughters about remaining true to themselves despite crushing pressure to conform."

—**Michelle Icard**, author of *Eight Setbacks That Can Make a Child a Success*

"*Restoring Our Girls* is the guide that daughters deserve to have parents read. Cathy Cassani Adams is an experienced and trustworthy guide, teaching us to listen, engage, and support our girls in such a way that they

can fearlessly and unquestioningly embody their most authentic selves. As a therapist, mother, and auntie, I am so grateful for this book."

—**Alexandra H. Solomon, PhD**, licensed clinical psychologist, faculty at Northwestern University, bestselling author of *Love Every Day*, and host of the podcast, *Reimagining Love*

"*Restoring Our Girls* is a gem of a book. Generation X, in particular, has worked hard to raise young women who know themselves better than we did, with the ultimate hope that they are able to blend an abiding self-love and a deep empathy for others to create an inner foundation that lasts a lifetime. This is no easy feat, and one that took many of us decades to integrate fully into our own lives. This book gives parents a blueprint for how it might be done with love, humor, embrace of paradox, respect for nuance, and real talk. The journey that Cathy highlights for us is often messy, but it's thorough and honest, and the rewards are great. Young girls who, from the beginning, develop a greater self-awareness and an acknowledgment of how their lives intersect with a big, beautiful world, eventually become women with the capacity to live more fully and joyfully in their own skin. I hope this book reaches the hands of many."

—**Annie Burnside**, author of *Soul to Soul Parenting* and *From Role to Soul*

"If you have girls in your life, you need this book! Cathy Cassani Adams understands how girls are struggling and has done the real work to understand what they need. *Restoring Our Girls* walks parents, caregivers, and anyone who has girls in their lives through real conversations and authentic communication that connects and heals. *Restoring Our Girls* gives a refreshing and wise perspective on how to navigate the unsettled waters of girlhood without talking down to either parents or girls—quite a feat! For girls everywhere I couldn't be happier that this book is in the world."

—**Hunter Clarke-Fields**, author of *Raising Good Humans* and creator of *Mindful Parenting*

RESTORING
OUR
GIRLS

Restoring Our Girls

How Real Conversations
Shape Our Daughters' Lives,
Help Them with Teen Challenges,
& Remind Them That They Matter

by

Cathy Cassani Adams, LCSW

MIAMI

Copyright © 2024 by Cathy Cassani Adams.
Published by Mango Publishing, a division of Mango Publishing Group, Inc.

Cover, Layout & Design: Megan Werner
Cover Photo: KereAktifGraphic / stock.adobe.com

Mango is an active supporter of authors' rights to free speech and artistic expression in their books. The purpose of copyright is to encourage authors to produce exceptional works that enrich our culture and our open society.

Uploading or distributing photos, scans or any content from this book without prior permission is theft of the author's intellectual property. Please honor the author's work as you would your own. Thank you in advance for respecting our author's rights.

For permission requests, please contact the publisher at:
Mango Publishing Group
5966 South Dixie Highway, Suite 300
Miami, FL 33143
info@mango.bz

For special orders, quantity sales, course adoptions and corporate sales, please email the publisher at sales@mango.bz. For trade and wholesale sales, please contact Ingram Publisher Services at customer.service@ingramcontent.com or +1.800.509.4887.

Restoring Our Girls: How Real Conversations Shape Our Daughters' Lives, Help Them with Teen Challenges, & Remind Them That They Matter

Library of Congress Cataloging-in-Publication number: has been requested
ISBN: (p) 978-1-68481-683-5 (e) 978-1-68481-684-2
BISAC category code FAM043000, FAMILY & RELATIONSHIPS / Life Stages / Teenagers

The information provided in this book is based on the research, insights, and experiences of the author. Every effort has been made to provide accurate and up-to-date information; however, neither the author nor the publisher warrants the information provided is free of factual error. This book is not intended to diagnose, treat, or cure any medical condition or disease, nor is it intended as a substitute for professional medical care. All matters regarding your health should be supervised by a qualified healthcare professional. The author and publisher disclaim all liability for any adverse effects arising out of or relating to the use or application of the information or advice provided in this book.

To my favorites, Todd, Jacey, Camryn, and Skylar.

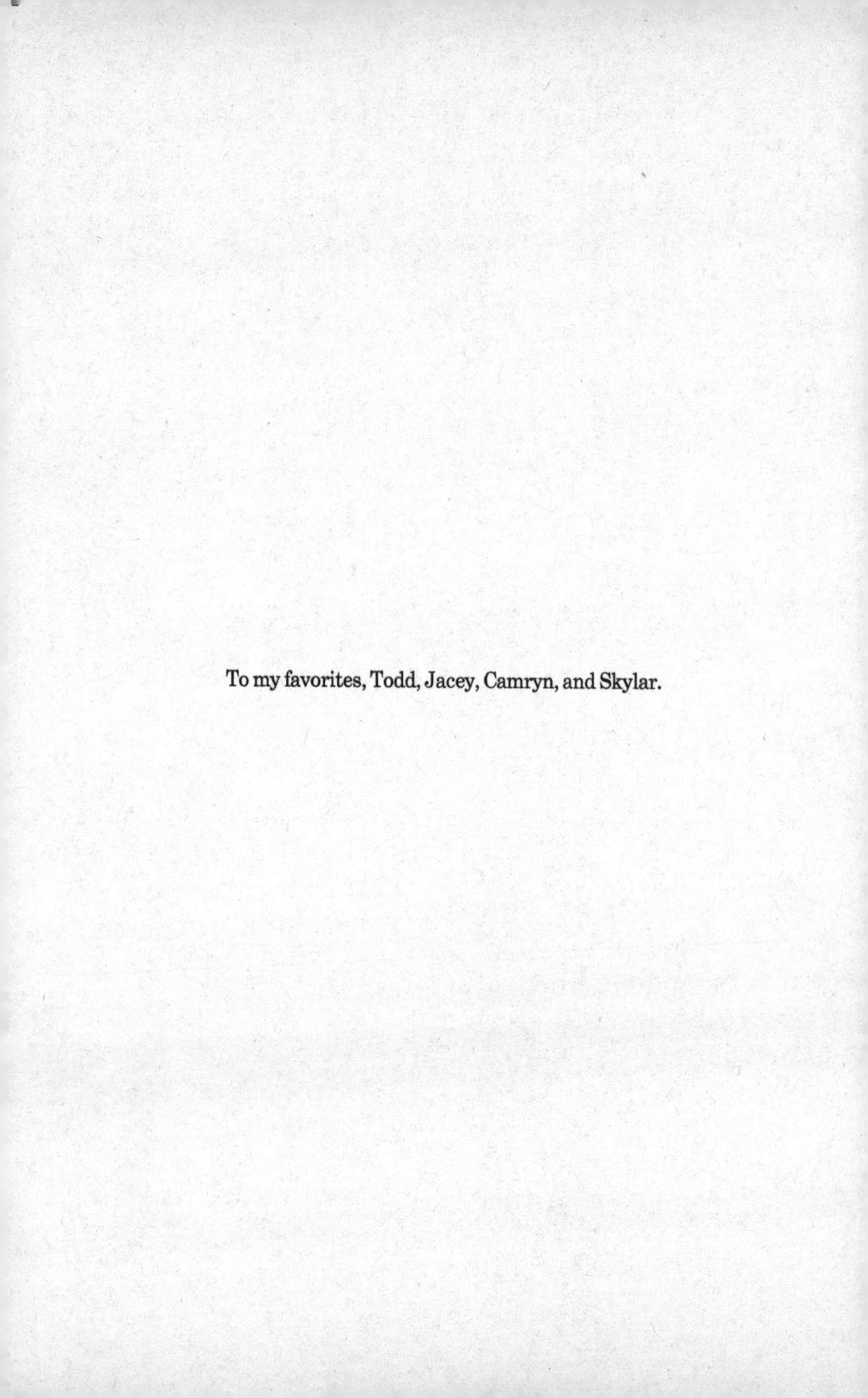

*what's the greatest lesson a woman should learn?
that since day one. she's already had everything
she needs within herself. it's the world that
convinced her she did not.*

—**rupi kaur**

TABLE OF CONTENTS

Foreword	12
A Note on Gender and Age	15
Introduction: Can You Please Tell My Parents This?	16
Chapter 1: Why Our Girls Need Real Conversations	23
Our Girls Are Struggling	28
Navigating a Complex Journey	33
Chapter 2: Why We Are Afraid of Real Conversations	38
Chapter 3: A Guide for Real Conversations	46
Widen Your Perspective	47
See Their Viewpoint	56
Encourage Critical Thinking	63
Eliminate These Phrases	79
Repair	87
Adapt	94
Lead	103
Be Light	112
Chapter 4: Real Things Girls Want You to Know	123
Know Me	124
Connect with Me	134
Support Me	148
Trust Me	161
Laugh with Me	169

Chapter 5: Real Stories from My Daughters	180
Expectation and Comparison	181
Appearance	189
Eating	195
Conclusion: Prioritize the Relationship	209
Acknowledgments	214
About the Author	217

Foreword

I've written and spoken quite a bit about the challenges our boys and young men are facing these days. But without a doubt, our girls and young women are suffering their own crises as well. Girls today are brilliant, possessing a striking degree of emotional intelligence, empathy, and self-awareness.

But their keen sense of self-awareness can drive what one young female client of mine calls *identity traffic*. Along with many of her peers, she describes all the internal identities she needs to keep track of daily: her identity with her parents, her siblings, her friends, her teachers and coaches and bosses.

And her online identity, which takes up far too much of her time and energy, while draining her sense of self-worth.

And finally, her identity with herself, someone she is not always comfortable facing.

With so much on her plate, a teenage girl today struggles to feel fully known by others and by herself. She needs to feel that she's important, that her life matters.

As a therapist who has worked with teenage girls for decades, I can tell you they have a need to be fully heard, and they need parents available to guide them through the myriad challenges of adolescence.

FOREWORD

Your daughters need your assistance to manage conflict with ease, to differentiate healthy vs. unhealthy relationships, and to make the right decisions for themselves in their complex and messy lives.

Some parents have suggested to me that their daughters neither want nor need to talk with them or hear from them.

But I assure you, they do.

She needs you to provide some sanctuary from all the noise she carries in her mind, help slow her thinking, ease her anxieties, and guide her through these times. The girls I've worked with often feel a deep sense of loneliness, a lack of feeling truly known. I find they long for real, meaningful discussion to meet their emotional needs, to feel known, connected, supported, trusted, and loved. The real conversations in this book will be your guide to understanding and acknowledging your girls, helping your daughters to feel whole in their complicated worlds.

And, at times, they need you to lend some perspective by bringing nuance and humor to their concerns. This book shines a light here as well.

I don't know anyone more appropriate to lead us in guiding our girls through these difficult years than Cathy Adams. When I have a question about how to guide one of the teenage girls I'm working with, Cathy is my immediate go-to expert colleague. Cathy is a brilliant leader, writer, speaker, educator, and therapist. And she comes to this particular work from a place of true *knowing*.

With her husband Todd, Cathy has raised three daughters herself, all among my favorite human beings on the planet. With them and so many others, I've seen Cathy practice the discussions, connections, acknowledgment, and empathy she describes in this book. I admire

RESTORING OUR GIRLS

Cathy's ability to strip the distractions and complexity of parenting girls down to simple, authentic, deeply empathic tools that really work.

Cathy *knows*. And she generously shares it all here in *Restoring Our Girls*.

This is a most important book at just the right moment. These are crucial, ever-changing, and confusing times for our girls and young women. Our effective guidance and availability are imperative. With just the right combination of wisdom, warmth, and humor, Cathy leads you toward truly, effectively restoring our girls to their most powerful, authentic selves.

The gift of *Restoring Our Girls* is already an integral component of my practice with girls and their parents. Keep this one close. I promise you'll find yourself referring to it often.

—**Dr. John Duffy**, author of *Rescuing Our Sons* and *Parenting the New Teen in the Age of Anxiety*

A Note on Gender and Age

Recognizing the uniqueness of each person, this book acknowledges that it cannot capture every aspect of the female experience, given the complexity and multifaceted nature of gender identity. Drawing from over twenty years of client experiences with girls from diverse backgrounds—including race, ethnicity, socioeconomic status, neurodiversity, gender and sexual identity—this book reflects commonly shared viewpoints of the female experience. It's unsurprising that there are plenty of universal experiences that transcend gender, where we can all find commonality and meaning.

I wrote this book as a Gen X woman (1965–1980), primarily working with Gen X moms, while raising and working with Gen Z girls (1997–2013), which makes the girls most referenced in this book between twelve and twenty-five years old. While the teenage years are known for their challenges, the real conversations discussed in the book may begin in preadolescence and continue beyond the teen years into the mid-twenties. And then, hopefully, beyond that, and into forever.

INTRODUCTION

Can You Please Tell My Parents This?

~~~~~~

The first time someone asked me to talk to their parents I was in second grade. My friend and I were putting away Matchbox cars, but we couldn't find the case where they belonged. We looked everywhere, but it was nowhere to be found, and my friend was getting increasingly panicked. Her parents were strict about cleanliness and organization, and because the cars belonged to her older sister, she knew that playing with them was a privilege that could be taken away.

I remember feeling that we hadn't done anything wrong here, we just couldn't locate the case. It felt quite reasonable to me. But I could also understand her fear—I had heard her parents yell at her for things that didn't feel fair or make sense, and I also knew I never wanted to disappoint my own parents, so in that way I could relate.

She asked me to go with her to talk to her parents and explain, so I did. This felt big—other people's parents were big—but I felt we could tell the truth and it would make sense. My friend started talking, but then stopped and looked at me, so I continued explaining the details of the lost case. I don't remember exactly what I said, or what her parents said, but I remember feeling like we were doing this right, we were solving this problem. It was big and uncomfortable, but confronting it openly and honestly was also the quickest path to the best outcome. I didn't know that for sure in second grade, but I do know it now.

Many other opportunities, challenges, and missteps, and a lot of formal education later, helped me validate the necessity of real conversations. I have built my life around the importance of real talks, as a therapist, podcaster, teacher, writer, and in my most vulnerable roles, as partner and parent. I have failed as much as I've succeeded, but personally and professionally, I've come to better decipher what people need and why they respond the way they do. I also spent a decade really diving into myself, figuring out why and how I stumbled in conversations and what I needed emotionally to handle them better. I applied these lessons to my everyday life, which for several decades has involved working with women and young women, and raising three daughters.

My hope is that, through real, sometimes difficult conversations, the girls we're raising today will have less to unlearn and more permission to know themselves and trust who they are. This means they'll have less to untangle as they get older, and they can be less self-critical, with fewer thoughts about not being good enough, needing to look better, worrying about others, needing to be less angry, and all the other myths we impose on girls.

As parents, therapists, and educators, we have considerable influence when it comes to nurturing girls' self-awareness and safeguarding their inner worlds. They will still be confronted by a culture and society that expect them to bow down and conform, but our ability to openly discuss and understand their experiences with them as they navigate these demands is what allows them to remain whole.

Navigating real conversations with our girls can feel daunting because it also requires facing messy and uncomfortable aspects of ourselves. Meaningful conversations necessitate valuing our views while recognizing our flaws—a paradoxical concept that isn't typically taught as we grow up. As young girls, we're told to fit in, accommodate, conform, and even acquiesce. Then growing up and maturing is all about questioning these expectations, unlearning layer upon layer to rediscover a clearer, more appreciative view of ourselves. This can take decades, and for some, it doesn't happen at all.

Why do we waste so much time learning only to have to painfully unlearn it later, and why do we continue this cycle as we raise this generation of girls? I've spent my career working with young girls and their parents, and despite the many changes in our culture, the struggle to communicate effectively with our daughters remains. Our persistence in imposing outdated expectations on them and our reluctance to question what might be harmful continue to be issues.

Gen Z has significantly more access to information and greater emotional awareness, but these advantages become drawbacks when it comes to interacting with their parents. Older generations struggle to understand these young girls; they didn't have the same opportunities or support to speak up and express themselves as girls do now. Pair that with a strong urge to make them conform to our beliefs, perspectives, and expectations for their future, and we can see where the conflict begins.

Everyone eventually faces a challenge to their outward identity, and for most of the Gen X moms I work with, this tends to show up as a midlife challenge. But for their daughters, it seems to be happening earlier and at a faster pace. They are being confronted with loss, grief, addiction, failure, or pain at an earlier stage, pushing them to reassess their understanding of reality.

CAN YOU PLEASE TELL MY PARENTS THIS?

These girls require assistance in processing what they are seeing and experiencing; they need genuine conversations, not superficial pleasantries that only appear clean and tidy on the surface. They need relationships with their parents that are trusting and supportive, rather than adversarial. Establishing an environment that embraces genuine conversations, approaches challenges with curiosity instead of shame, and welcomes our less glamorous aspects with understanding creates the foundation they are seeking.

For years, girls have confided in me, sharing their struggles and wishing they could be more accepting of themselves, and that life didn't hurt so much. They want to trust who they are, but they've learned they can't—not because they're incapable, but because of the messages they've absorbed. They want to talk to their parents but are afraid they will be met with a rejection that reinforces their pain. What they need is understandable and what they want is relatable—the hope is that parents can understand and relate, too.

Some parents do understand, but many do not. In my work with parents, I hear how much they are struggling with their own unresolved issues from their past, still finding it hard to reconcile their own pain. Because of this, it's difficult to have enough clarity or space to relate to what their daughters are going through, or to try something different when it comes to parenting. They feel attached to a certain model or theory, often similar to the way they were raised, that focuses more on changing their daughters than on questioning themselves.

Participating in genuine conversations and attentively listening to our daughters necessitates being open to change. This could involve seeing them from a different perspective or reexamining our own worldview. It's challenging—I'm a parent to three daughters myself, so I understand why parents feel uneasy and overwhelmed. I can relate to the reluctance to let go of what we believe works, or how we think life should unfold.

RESTORING OUR GIRLS

But the effort is worth it if it means establishing meaningful relationships with our girls and reducing the pain they experience and inflict upon themselves. This is reinforced when girls are sharing so vulnerably and bravely—then one of them will jokingly, or even earnestly, say to me, "Can you please tell my parents this?"

"This" essentially means:

- Will you help them understand who I am so they will *know me*?
- Will you ask them not to shame me or judge me, and instead *connect with me*?
- Will you help them become better listeners and *support me*?
- Will you remind them that I am doing my best and to *trust me*?
- Will you tell them to take life less seriously and *laugh with me*?

As a professor, I've taught introductory social work classes to predominantly female college students for over a decade, and every week there is a young woman who lingers after class to seek advice on bringing up sensitive topics with her parents, like choosing a major that goes against her parents' preferences, sharing academic setbacks or missed internship opportunities, or even revealing a pregnancy, an experience with sexual assault, or involvement in an abusive relationship.

They long for connection and understanding from their parents, but based on past experience, they anticipate conversations going badly, tensions rising, and communication breaking down. This makes it hard for them to share anything without a careful, thought-out plan, which leads to them experiencing overwhelming anxiety as they even consider it.

Even when we are open to conversations with our girls, there are inevitable obstacles. We come to each discussion with so many defenses, easily taking offense or feeling triggered—and that's just our side of the conversation. Our girls are dealing with similar challenges, but with less emotional maturity. All of this makes it increasingly hard to hear each other and connect.

Our struggles to communicate effectively with our daughters don't mean we don't love them enough; in fact, our emotionality, fear, or worry is there because we are trying to show them how much we do love them, but our methods end up backfiring. Parents I talk to typically find it easier to communicate with their nieces or their kids' friends about difficult issues, but when it comes to their own daughters, they very quickly get flooded and overwhelmed.

Our love for our daughters intensifies the pressure, leading us to believe that, to love them, we have to exert force, coerce, and maintain control—but these are the very things that hurt communication and create disconnection. The purpose of this book is to heighten our self-awareness and bridge the communication gap with our daughters. To engage with them in a way that reduces reactivity on our part and creates a greater sense of understanding for them.

People often ask why therapy is effective, and while there are numerous factors, a key element is the ability to verbalize our thoughts and emotions, share our experiences, and have them witnessed and validated by another person. Parents don't need to be therapists, but they can learn from this insight. Creating space for our daughters to freely express themselves, to feel heard and understood without judgment, creates a sense of grounding within them. Simply listening provides reassurance and validates their emotional well-being. Sometimes, this is all they need.

How our girls communicate with us influences how they express themselves elsewhere, and our actions set the standard for what they perceive as normal. The ability to have conversations will go way beyond

RESTORING OUR GIRLS

our home; they shape how our girls will interact with the world and develop their own adult relationships.

This book is for parents, educators, therapists, and any adult who is interested, but it's also for all the girls who have asked me to talk to their parents. Maybe your girls will come across this book and share it with you, or maybe you'll come across it and share it with them. The goal is to start a conversation and keep it open and ongoing. It's about trusting each other enough to communicate with dignity and humility, to have the conversations that are difficult, but then lead to the intimacy and connection we all deserve.

CHAPTER 1

Why Our Girls Need Real Conversations

The perspectives shared in this book stem from my years of close collaboration with girls and women. The stories are inspired by the invaluable lessons learned from girls, but their insights and wisdom will often feel universally relatable, speaking to everyone, regardless of gender or relationship dynamics.

My work has always centered around talking to girls, beginning with my role as a therapist in a partial hospitalization setting—where I connected with girls from all over the city of Chicago—to my work as a college professor, primarily teaching Latina and Black young women aspiring to be social workers. I teach sex education to girls in parochial schools and lead self-empowerment sessions for girls in schools across Chicagoland, and I created and facilitated a self-empowerment curriculum for adolescent girls called Be U.

I facilitate an international virtual parenting community and host both live and virtual women's circles, and in my private therapy practice, I specialize in working with women and their daughters. But it's my role as a mother to three daughters that provides me with the most real and intimate understanding of what girls and their friends are asking for.

This book brings together what I've gathered from young women—their common concerns, hopes, and dreams. It reveals what they wish their parents knew, how they wish they could communicate, and what they are hoping for in life. It also explores why they often feel so depressed, so not enough, and so anxious. Their needs are not always gender-specific—like everyone else, they just want to feel understood and valued, to know that they are seen and loved. Whether you're a parent or not, there's a lot to learn here about how to better communicate and connect more deeply with all the people we care about.

While girls' fundamental human needs are indeed universal, their cultural experiences are very different. There is a different reality when you are raised in a society shaped by male perspectives. From the history taught in schools to the music, movies, and heroes celebrated, the cultural tilt toward the male experience is reality. While the arrow seems to be pointed toward equality, every step forward—like the #MeToo movement—is met with a step back—like the overturning of *Roe v. Wade*—making balance feel elusive.

As I write this, Harvey Weinstein's criminal conviction in New York—a landmark case in the #MeToo movement—was just overturned, leading to the need for a new trial or a dismissal of charges. Prosecutors established his sexual misconduct by offering testimony from multiple accusers, and the courts decided that including so many voices had potentially biased the jury.

On the same day, Idaho is defending its near-total abortion ban before the Supreme Court, which doesn't include exceptions to protect the health of pregnant women. The state law prohibits nearly all abortions except in cases of imminent maternal death, refusing to even consider situations where the woman's health is at risk. Weeks later, the Senate moved a bill to codify protections for women accessing contraception and another bill to protect in vitro fertilization (IVF), but they both failed, with only two Republicans—both female—voting yes.

It can be incredibly challenging for women and young women to digest the news every day, given the prevailing message that appears to encourage our silence, smallness, and insignificance, with a small group of powerful men making decisions for our health and well-being. The stark contrast between the stories we're told about our progress, freedom, and safety, and the actual realities we face, creates a profound sense of cognitive dissonance.

Even in the face of this challenging environment, girls demonstrate a remarkable capacity to adapt within the culture. They have good role models, as many amazing women have figured out how to survive and thrive in a world that was not built for them. Many girls work hard to advance women's rights while also developing an ability to understand, not only their own viewpoint, but also the viewpoints of others, especially the male perspective.

Girls are taught about historical figures, like Abraham Lincoln, Albert Einstein, and Martin Luther King Jr., who are hailed as heroes, while pop culture icons such as Luke Skywalker, Harry Potter, and Tony Stark/Iron Man are celebrated for their influence. Male musicians like Elvis Presley, Bruce Springsteen, Freddy Mercury, and Prince are revered as musical legends and for their greatness—but despite achieving comparable or even higher levels of success, women like Taylor Swift and Beyoncé face obstacles to being recognized as "great." Swift is often dismissed as catering only to teenage girls, while Beyoncé's artistry is deemed too complex or unconventional, which can also be easily attributed to racial biases.

RESTORING OUR GIRLS

Male sports get significant more attention and support in our culture, with bigger audiences, more money, and more media coverage. This not only affects how people see athleticism, but also keeps gender differences and inequalities alive. In 2024, women's NCAA basketball—particularly the achievements of players like Caitlin Clark and Angel Reese, who received notable media attention—attracted even larger audiences than the men's college basketball. This was exciting, but notably rare. The sportscasters themselves expressed astonishment at the opportunity to discuss women's basketball to such an extent, acknowledging the typical underpromotion and minimal coverage of women's sports by most sports media outlets.

In a culture shaped by male influence, feminism—which is grounded in the pursuit of equality and justice for all genders—is necessary. Championing women's rights doesn't detract from opportunities for men; it's an opportunity for a more balanced and inclusive societal and cultural experience. Gender equality isn't just fair, it builds economies, with research showing that closing the gender gap improves economic conditions. It's not about turning against men or assigning blame; it's an educational awareness opportunity, a way to unite and acknowledge the strengths of a society that values and benefits from both the masculine and feminine.

When discussing patriarchy—which is a system created and predominantly led by men—we don't need to vilify masculinity or overlook its range and complexity. Individual men do not need to feel offended or blamed. It's recognizing that our world and experiences are predominantly shaped by male perspectives, and that meaning comes from creations and stories crafted by men. It's the air we breathe and the water we swim in, and as women, we are tasked with figuring out how to fit into this framework. Cue America Ferrera's *Barbie* monologue.

WHY OUR GIRLS NEED REAL CONVERSATIONS

When discussing feminism or patriarchy and observing the reactions they elicit, it becomes obvious that some segments of society have framed these words negatively. Resistance to these words suggests either a broader discomfort with equality, or, I think more often, a misunderstanding of the definitions and their implications. I can sense a shift in the room, a discomfort or quietness, when I bring up feminism or discuss the challenges of living in a patriarchy (which affects all genders). Are you feeling it right now as you read this?

Our hesitance to address gender disparities highlights the discomfort within our societal norms. This is why girls often find themselves walking a tightrope—they know they will be rewarded for conforming to societal expectations, they know they are supposed to challenge norms, and they also know they'll be criticized if they step out of line. It's a delicate balance—one that leaves girls feeling uncertain about where they belong or how much freedom they really have to be themselves.

There's a strong urge to control women's bodies and choices in our society, evident in the recent assaults on reproductive rights and bodily autonomy. Laws and social norms are shaped primarily by white men in positions of power, forcing women and marginalized groups little choice but to conform or revolt. We're trying to figure out who we are and stand up for our rights when things aren't fair, but we feel torn inside from juggling the conflicting societal pressures to just "be nice" and get along. Plus, the workload and caregiving expectations we already experience can leave us with insufficient time to make a substantial impact or difference.

This book is structured to first address problems like these, focusing on the reasons our girls are struggling right now and why real conversations are necessary. It then explores our adult fears about having real conversations with our girls and offers a practical guide for improving our communication skills and ability to connect. It concludes with the real things girls say and why certain issues affect them, and ways we can avoid land mines in conversations and alleviate their concerns. The final section features stories from my own daughters, ages twenty-one, twenty, and seventeen, each sharing a personal struggle. They recount their experiences and I offer how I, as their mom, experienced their experiences.

Although this book will address challenges, its primary goal is not to comment on every obstacle that girls and women encounter. Instead, it focuses on communication and connection, and the barriers that hinder success in these areas. I will highlight some societal issues that present obvious obstacles to emphasize that girls' experiences are complex, nuanced, and individual. There's a whole mess of factors that contribute to their present-day challenges, and a lot of it isn't their doing or within their control—it's just the cultural norms they were born into.

OUR GIRLS ARE STRUGGLING

Our girls are navigating the pressures and coping mechanisms of their time, sharing struggles with cutting, eating disorders, alcohol and drug abuse, vaping, cyberbullying, loneliness, and concerns about their mental well-being, overall safety, and reproductive autonomy. Each girl has a unique story, and her challenges not only warrant being heard and understood, but also demand individualized, focused attention. We also need to recognize that, whatever the challenges may be, they are not just about her, but are part of a larger systemic issue.

During my work with girls in inpatient and partial hospitalization programs, they were engaged and eager to learn and shift unhealthy behaviors, but upon returning home to an unchanged environment, they usually reverted to old patterns and cycled back through the program. Families operate like teams, where everyone's actions affect everyone else, and individual issues need to be addressed as family issues, prompting everyone to seek new ways to communicate and interact.

According to the Centers for Disease Control and Prevention (CDC), from 2021 data, nearly three out of five teen girls experience persistent feelings of sadness or hopelessness, a figure double that of boys. This is the highest level reported in the past decade. While the pandemic contributed to this issue, mental health challenges among girls were already on the rise. Between 2010 and 2019, cases of depression among girls doubled, and there has been a steady increase in concerning behaviors such as self-harm, suicide attempts, and deaths by suicide.

Parents and the media anxiously question whether girls are truly facing more challenges than earlier generations, or if they are simply becoming more open about discussing their difficulties. The answer is yes, and yes. Girls are more open to sharing, but when they don't yet have the tools to adequately express their needs, or there is no one who is willing to listen and understand, they are left feeling the same, or often worse, because their cries for help are disregarded or misunderstood.

When they're not getting noticed, they might push hard to be seen, which can be exhausting and risky, sometimes causing them to drift away from their family. Alternatively, they could end up stuck in a cycle of hospitalizations or other interventions. They might also end up neglecting their own needs and simply conforming, which can lead to a loss of identity and inner turmoil in the future.

They are confronted with more complex challenges than any previous generation, growing up in an increasingly consumer-driven culture that demands conformity to an ever-changing ideal. They are confronted with rapidly evolving technology, rising societal pressures, and shifting cultural norms with unattainable expectations for appearance, achievement, and behavior.

They face academic pressure, unreasonable beauty standards, sexual violence, fear of climate change, threats of gun violence, and obstacles to accessing contraception and asserting bodily autonomy. They rely on a social media landscape filled with trolling and online hate, and if you are a person of color and/or a member of the LGBTQ+ community, just add even more challenge and political volatility to the mix. Let's just say they are struggling to hold on to their true selves, especially when so much of their identity is intertwined with this online environment.

Social media intensifies the pressure girls feel, offering a platform where lives are showcased and compared, ultimately resulting in feelings of inadequacy and self-doubt. The dependency on social media and the constant exposure to curated images and idealized lives results in impractical expectations about success and happiness. The pressure to conform to these standards gradually erodes their sense of self and undermines their ability to be real.

With all the negative effects of social media, there are a few positive aspects, particularly for girls. Social media provides a valuable platform for self-expression, learning, and virtual friendships, and the online community can at times be a comforting resource, offering an outlet and a source of stability when girls need it most.

Social media is for sure a mixed bag, functioning as a fantastic resource that can change lives, while also being an experience that can lead to exclusion and increased loneliness. We are forced to contend with it because it's firmly rooted in our culture, but face-to-face interactions with those who sincerely care about our well-being are, and will always be, the greatest source of comfort, offering the highest potential for positive shifts and a greater regard for ourselves and our sense of belonging. That's why the goal is to establish a culture in the home where conversations, questions, and even disagreements are encouraged, allowing us to normalize and address needs as they arise.

Having real conversations and actively listening helps young women trust that the adults in their lives are supportive allies. As therapist and author Terry Real says, there is no such thing as "working on a relationship"—to nurture a relationship, we need to focus on ourselves individually within the relationship. As parents, we take responsibility for our part by practicing availability, vulnerability, and, most importantly, humility, to create an atmosphere of safety and trust. Then our girls can rely on us without worrying that they will be subjected to ridicule or shame.

Having open and honest conversations with young girls about their lives and the world can be uncomfortable and difficult, so it's important to remember that *we don't have to have all the answers, just the willingness to participate*. By simply engaging in real conversations, we encourage our girls to think critically, ponder, and empathize. Real conversations empower our girls to:

1. Recognize and share what they feel.
2. Approach and manage conflict maturely and confidently.
3. Ask for help.
4. Communicate effectively.
5. Differentiate between helpful and harmful relationships.
6. Discern and investigate nuance and paradox.
7. Practice self-awareness and critical thinking.
8. Embrace life's imperfections and messiness.

While the advice shared in these chapters can be helpful to individuals of all genders and ages, young women face distinctive challenges as they navigate their physical, psychological, sexual, and emotional development. The lives of girls and women are distinct, and my goal is to provide insights and strategies that demonstrate a personal and comprehensive understanding of their unique needs.

I'm married to a man who leads an international men's group focused on connection and healthy masculinity, providing me with insights into the genuine challenges boys and men encounter in today's world. Currently, there's significant attention on these issues, with numerous statistics indicating that men are increasingly dealing with feeling lost, lonely, overlooked, and undervalued in society.

These shifts have influenced our political culture and have led to social isolation, incel behavior (young men without romantic partners despite desiring them, often resulting in misogyny and blaming women for perceived failures), online trolling, and outward displays of anger and violence, frequently involving gun violence. A significant portion of this aggression and violence is directed at women, highlighting the interconnected nature of our needs and well-being. We need to prioritize understanding men and boys alongside women and girls—it's not an "either/or" scenario, but a "both/and" approach.

Women and girls are the demographic I know, study, work with, teach, and happen to be raising as the mother of three daughters. My personal and professional experience working with girls and women offers me unique access to their perspectives. If you also have sons, I recommend seeking out similar information specific to their needs. I personally recommend Dr. John Duffy's book, *Rescuing Our Sons*, and the nonprofit organization my husband founded, MenLiving.org.

WHY OUR GIRLS NEED REAL CONVERSATIONS

NAVIGATING A COMPLEX JOURNEY

When my oldest daughter was thirteen, she and her best friend decided to walk downtown for dinner. They dressed up, put on makeup, and made it an event—a chance to do something older girls do. It was a significant step for them, going out alone. They wanted to appear older, and they succeeded. I wanted to warn them to be careful, to pay close attention to each other and their surroundings. I felt like Forrest Gump before he puts his son on a bus, wanting to warn him about everything that could happen, but then realizing it's best to simply say, "I love you." So, I just waved goodbye, and told them to call if they had any issues or needed a ride.

When they returned from dinner, they had so many stories to share. While at the restaurant, some college guys had invited them to join their table. The girls declined, but struggled not to smile and laugh with embarrassment, which encouraged the guys to continue. The guys persisted, but the waitress intervened, advising the guys to back off while staying close to my daughter's table, encouraging them to ignore the guys' behavior. Then, on their way home, the girls encountered catcalling for the first time, with not just one, but two cars honking at them.

I didn't even know where to start; so many issues, so many real-world things to process. We discussed the fun of dressing up and feeling attractive, but also how it can draw unwanted attention. We talked about the thrill of being noticed by boys, but also stressed the importance of being cautious and aware of potential dangers. We discussed how women often look out for each other, mostly because they've had their own experiences of needing protection or support.

We covered as much as they could handle that night, and now my daughter is twenty-one, and the conversation has never ended. Her recent trip to Italy brought up similar lessons about safety, the advantages of having a man to travel with or have in her social group, and the cultural differences around flirting and catcalling. This conversation will always be ongoing—it's an enduring part of the female experience.

Growing up as a girl means facing inherent contradictions, where moments of joy and risk often collide. As a mother of three girls, I don't want to scare them about the world, and like any parent, I want them to feel courageous and empowered. But they have to stay aware of their surroundings, be cautious about who they trust, and avoid being in certain situations alone. They are simultaneously tasked with challenging the cultural conditioning that dictates they must always be nice and accommodating.

Recently, my daughter bought my husband a sticker for his computer featuring Ferdinand, the bull who prefers peace over fighting, sniffing a flower. Next to the picture, it says, "Let Boys Be Sweet." I love this sticker, but I also think we need one with Meg from *A Wrinkle in Time* or Jo from *Little Women* that says, "Let Girls Be Angry."

Our daughters are expected to be everything at once—decisive yet caring, autonomous yet collaborative, self-assured yet modest, daring yet cautious, empowered yet considerate, accomplished yet affable, self-sufficient yet caring. I get exhausted thinking about it. This relentless pursuit of meeting everyone's needs leaves them feeling overwhelmed, untethered, and constantly striving for unattainable ideals.

Our girls get contradictory messages about how to treat their bodies, starting with hyper-insistence that they should fixate on how they look, while simultaneously scolding them when they become obsessed with their appearance. They are told to embrace body positivity or body neutrality, regardless of size, but the social media expectations and the BMI chart tell them they are failing.

WHY OUR GIRLS NEED REAL CONVERSATIONS

Every day on social media, millions of girls share their OOTD (outfit of the day) and extend an invitation to GRWM (get ready with me), setting the stage for our girls to compare how they look, dress, or take care of their skin and hair. At some point, even my TikTok algorithm picked up the OOTD trend, and I caught myself thinking, *Do I need more bracelets? They seem to be back in style. And what about the shoes all these girls are hyping...should I get a pair?*

It's too easy to believe that we need more, or that we aren't enough, when we so easily see what others have. We can remind our daughters that social media influencers receive products to promote and profit from, but this doesn't stop them from feeling like they don't have enough, or like they aren't enough. The truth is, telling girls, or boys, to stop comparing is futile; instead, we can help them recognize why they compare, consider what they genuinely want, and process the reality behind having and needing more.

What lies beneath the desire to have things is the belief that the people who have things are happier. They look happier, and they tell us they are happier. As we get older, we understand the consumerism and placating that lie behind these messages, but our kids don't yet understand that they are being targeted for profit. Having stuff doesn't decrease insecurity, and sometimes the person who has the most stuff and needs to show it off to the world has the deepest self-loathing.

What I share with my daughters, and any girl I'm working with, is that everyone is struggling with something. The person who appears to "have it all" is often attempting to relieve pain through the acquiring of things. As a therapist, I have worked with so many girls and families from all different socioeconomic levels, and I can tell you that the ones who seem to have the most often feel the worst. They exude a persona of having it all, but their persona is a mask to guard against what they are feeling inside.

One conversation with our kids, or even a few, will not change this. It takes time and experience to recognize comparison culture, and it takes time and experience for our kids to recognize their self-worth. It's our job to lay the foundation and speak about it openly and honestly. Your girls may not initially agree, or may think you don't understand, but as they continue to live and be confronted with choices or viewpoints, they will keep your voice as the most trusted option to consider.

Girls are told that with hard work and sacrifice, they can be leaders, but they are met with gender bias and resistance when it comes to equal pay and advancement. They live in a society where one out of every six women has been sexually assaulted. Instead of being protected, they are blamed for what they wear or for not remembering all the details of a highly traumatic, brain-altering experience.

Girls are told to use their voices, to speak up and ask for help, but when they step forward, they are accused of being liars, dramatic, or selfish. Our daughters live in a constant paradox of existence, and to navigate it, they need the opportunity to acknowledge and discuss their experiences. They need a space where the people they care about the most will listen, validate, and help process the injustices they encounter.

When we are asked, we can also share our own life experiences, and demonstrate the importance of openly discussing topics that shaped our identity and perception of the world. In the parent-child dynamic, we are the leaders, so it's our job to continually find creative ways to discuss what's uncomfortable and uncover patterns that block us from doing so.

We can become more attuned to our girls by noticing when they are struggling, confused, or uncertain, like when their Instagram posts are filled with pictures of fun and joy, but we know they aren't really feeling what they are sharing. Difficult conversations require an ability to imagine the burden our girls experience, to take off our adult glasses and view the world as a teen who feels pressure to share these posts, to answer every Snap, to engage with TikTok, to do as others do. To ask them to "get over the pressure" lacks self-awareness and will be perceived as hypocritical. Are you over the pressure? Are any of us?

Our ability to listen and understand is how they find their center; their ability to trust their choices is how they become responsible and effective adults. When our daughters are at home, they long to set down the pressure and be themselves—not the selves we think they should be, or who other kids appear to be, but their true selves, who experience a slew of ever-changing emotions and a desire to connect with something meaningful.

Our girls want us to get better at just listening so they can open up without feeling like they always have to defend themselves or explain everything. They just want to relax with us and trust we won't judge them like the rest of the world does. They don't need us panicking about their grades, outfit, or social life. They genuinely want to feel safe, not like they're always under a spotlight. To help them find that comfort, we should consider giving them some breathing room by not sharing their lives on our social media, or at least by asking permission before we do.

With all the contradictory expectations our girls experience, they struggle to know who they are, and we may have difficulty seeing the girl standing in front of us. The one who has her own needs and goals, and the one who may be struggling or in pain. The one who may want something completely different than what we are expecting, and the only one who knows what's best for her.

CHAPTER 2

Why We Are Afraid of Real Conversations

~~~~~~

My sixteen-year-old daughter wanted to know why she was happy in the morning, but so annoyed by the end of the day. She asked why sometimes she feels like she can handle things, and other times, life feels too overwhelming. She wanted to know which perspective was real, or which version of reality she should trust.

I told her, in my best therapist voice, that *our perspectives are always changing, usually because of what's happening now or because of our past experiences and future worries…and that every emotion has wisdom, each offering guidance…* She cut me off to say, "So it will always feel like this? Even when I'm your age?"

I wanted to tell her, no, of course not. That as soon as she gets older, things will smooth out and happiness will become the primary feeling. I wanted to tell her that, in the next couple years, things will begin to make perfect sense, and that if she's just willing to hang in there, all her anxiety will fade, and she'll see herself and the world with such clarity. I

WHY WE ARE AFRAID OF REAL CONVERSATIONS

wanted to tell her that the discomfort she feels is fleeting, almost unreal, and that with age, she will know true peace.

But of course, I didn't, because it's not true. It might have been what she wanted to hear, but it wasn't genuine, and in the long run, it wouldn't have been helpful. Instead, I affirmed that her emotions will indeed always be ever-changing, and yes, unfortunately, she will continue to feel the anxiety of life.

But I also said that, while she can't totally rid herself of the discomfort, she will, over time, learn to notice, accept, and sometimes even let it all go—and that through this process, she will come to know herself on a much deeper level.

She stared, took a deep breath, raised her eyebrows, and sighed out a long "Okaaaay..." before heading upstairs to her room.

Naturally, it would be far more comforting—for both of us—if I could simply assure her with a cheery, "Hang tight, everything will magically fall into place soon enough!" There's a bit of truth in that sentiment, but it's not the full picture. It's like painting life with broad strokes and avoiding all the messy details. We need to learn how to navigate life's messiness, so it's essential to leave room for complexity and nuance in our conversations with our girls.

We need to normalize their connection to and trust in their inner world, and help them ground it in a realistic life perspective. Life is too complex for simple solutions, tropes, or absolutes, especially when our goal is to help our girls navigate life effectively. We aren't characters in a movie where we sit across from our girls at a table and deliver profound life lessons; they absorb life's lessons through ordinary, everyday conversations. They learn by observing how we interact and relate to our day-to-day experiences.

Real and profound conversations may feel like they don't fit into our busy schedules, but they don't always require extra time, and even when they do, they save us more time in the long run. The ability to start with humility, curiosity, and a willingness to keep conversations open and flowing decreases the likelihood of misunderstandings and disconnection that can take years to untangle. We are also presented the opportunity to discuss the world in a more multidimensional way, acknowledging paradox (acknowledging that pain can be both terrible and enlightening), encouraging critical thinking (questioning the source and validity of information), and promoting empathy (considering differing perspectives beyond their own experiences).

Engaging in more open-ended and ongoing conversations alleviates the pressure of a singular "sex talk" or a monumental discussion about weed or depression. Rather than trying to establish a single, high-stakes moment with our daughters, we can weave dynamic discussions into our daily lives.

I work with women, mostly mothers, who tell me what they wish they had had when they were growing up, why they felt silenced, what hurt them, why they needed more talks, support, and understanding. They openly share their sadness or longing with me; they express how their partners fail to show up for them in a way that makes them feel loved, or how their kids disrespect them or overlook everything they do to keep the household running smoothly. They feel incredibly alone in their experiences and yearn for more from their lives.

When I ask what their partner or kids say when they express what they need, I hear some version of this: "Well, I haven't told them. I don't know what I would say, and it wouldn't make a difference anyway."

We know we need something different, but we don't trust ourselves to speak it. We realize we're unhappy but struggle to pinpoint the

WHY WE ARE AFRAID OF REAL CONVERSATIONS

exact reasons why. We know we want more, but either believe we don't deserve it or think we would never have access to it anyway. We fear disappointment and rejection, so instead of having our hearts broken—again—we choose to do what we always do, because at least it's predictable and consistent.

This is tough, and if you're feeling it, you're not alone. Today, there's immense pressure on moms to confront their own pasts, identify what they missed out on, ask for what they need, and then pave a new path for their daughters. It can feel like doubling the workload on top of an already doubled workload. And if we become more self-aware or start speaking our minds, we often face questions about why we're changing things or causing disruption. Women's journeys are acceptable only if they don't inconvenience anyone else.

Still, we have to dare to envision and believe that we deserve something different, that we are worthy of what we need. This is how we rediscover ourselves, and how we empower our daughters to do the same. Change will be a gradual process, requiring us to make small adjustments and requests to see real progress.

We miss out on understanding what our daughters need when we haven't taken the time to figure out what we need. Unless we've done some soul-searching through therapy, coaching, or simply practicing some kind of self-awareness, we are usually in the dark about the energy and experiences we bring to our parenting. Some of us believe that we are supposed to give our kids the exact same childhood we had, or we go to the other extreme and swear we'll be the complete opposite of our own parents. But either way, it's still about us—our own past and the experiences we had or didn't have.

Parenting is about supporting our children in becoming themselves. If we are constantly stuck in what we did or didn't get, consciously or unconsciously, we miss the opportunity to truly be present for our girls. Notice how, a page or two ago, I mentioned the importance of focusing on ourselves, and now I'm saying we shouldn't focus too much on ourselves? This is an example of a both/and situation, a negotiation with complexity, an understanding of holding two truths at once. Our ability to wrestle with this and learn how to toggle back and forth in our conversations with our girls teaches them to do the same. Through our conversational practices, we demonstrate how to navigate complexity.

Being a parent means we will inevitably have times of overload, which creates a great opportunity to start advocating for our needs or, at the very least, to recognize and pay attention to them. It's a chance to question the culture and our conditioning, to acknowledge our history and current situation, and to treat ourselves with care. If we don't, our discomfort and disharmony will be sensed by our daughters. Not because we intend to harm or unload on them, but because communication is not just words—it's energy. Our girls can tell when we're unhappy and unsure of ourselves. Believe me, they know.

The good news is that we don't have to pretend to feel good all the time. We get to be real people, feeling our emotions, experiencing what all humans do. But we also need to demonstrate an ability to take care of ourselves in difficult times. Teaching our girls to prioritize themselves and their well-being is primarily done through role-modeling. We can't ask them to do something that we ourselves are unwilling to do, or feel undeserving of doing.

We are adults raising children, so it's our job to take care of ourselves and pay attention to our pain and history so our girls don't have to bear the brunt of our unmet needs. If we don't, our daughters may feel the need to live out our dreams or take care of us, leaving them to naturally lose track of themselves—and the cycle continues. Attempting to impose our childhood onto our children will inevitably not fit properly, and at the same time, hiding or repressing our childhood completely creates a noticeable silence or gaping hole. Again, we need to practice striking a balance between not burdening our kids with all our history and pain, and not keeping secrets that confuse them and shut them out.

The expectation of every generation is that we evolve—that we allow ourselves to be in this space and time and recognize that our childhood was a different space and time. Our parents did what they could with what they had—they made choices based on their situation, history, trauma, and societal expectations. Now it's our opportunity to do the same, but ideally with heightened awareness and emotional competence.

This is a lifelong practice, a continuous journey, where seeking professional support is always beneficial. I have personally experienced the value of therapy in my own life, from the early days of motherhood and dealing with the heartbreak of miscarriages, to navigating through periods of depression, heightened anxiety, and coping with chronic migraines. Therapy has also been instrumental in helping me grieve the health struggles and eventual deaths of my parents, as well as adjusting to my daughters growing up and becoming adults. Even during the ordinary challenges of everyday life, therapy has provided me with much-needed support and guidance.

I know I need this support because parenting is both a role and a relationship. The role encompasses our responsibilities, but it's the relationship that makes the responsibilities manageable, even engaging. When we overly prioritize our role and neglect the relationship, our daughters trust us less, struggle to hear us, and find it challenging to rely on us for emotional support, often fighting against us instead.

If we're emotionally unavailable, because our daughters perceive us as too busy, judgmental, or intimidating, our girls are left to navigate challenges alone or forced to rely on their peers. Right now, in the current political, social, technological and emotional climate, things are hard, and our girls need help shoring up their insides. They need to know they can come to us when they are overwhelmed by the mix of adult issues flooding through their devices and permeating their culture. They have plenty of people telling them what to do and why they should be different (just ask them, they will tell you). We don't need to join that choir. We get to be their support system, advocate, and reality-checker.

This is not coddling; this is relationship-building. In a healthy relationship, we tell the truth, we share our concerns, we offer feedback. We confront conflicts head-on, sometimes needing to deliver tough messages—saying no, discussing sensitive topics, or addressing harmful behaviors. But these conversations become much more manageable when built on a foundation of trust and support. When our girls know we stand by them, they feel safe to be their authentic selves and ask for what they need. Without that trust, they may nod along and tell us they are okay, but deep down, they're concealing their true feelings to avoid our judgment and their shame.

In my work with women in midlife, I still see them grappling with their relationships with their mothers, even if their mothers have already passed away. It's a journey most of us will undertake, even if our experiences with our moms were generally positive. But by making our relationship with our daughters a priority when they are young, we leave less of a mess to deal with as they age. We can establish healthy communication, take responsibility for things that are ours, and break some harmful family patterns. We can focus on who we really are individually and as family, rather than waste our energy trying to manage how others perceive us.

Remember that brief conversation with my sixteen-year-old about her feeling confused and whether she would always feel this way, even at my age? She came home from school the next day and said she'd heard

WHY WE ARE AFRAID OF REAL CONVERSATIONS

something in Chemistry that reminded her of our discussion. She said they were discussing relative humidity, and how in the summer, high humidity prevents sweat from evaporating easily, causing us to feel hot, while in winter, the very same humidity level makes us feel chilly, as the moisture in the air cools us down. The humidity percentage stays constant, but its impact changes with the season.

It was my turn to say, "Okaaay..." as I initially struggled to grasp the connection, but she explained that she saw a parallel between the way humidity feels different depending on the season, and the way fluctuating emotions feel different depending on age and maturity. It wasn't a perfect comparison, but that didn't matter. She was clearly contemplating, assimilating, or at least acknowledging our conversation, and so, of course, we kept talking. We discussed until she ran out of steam and once again headed up to her room.

CHAPTER 3

A Guide for Real Conversations

~~~~~~~

Real Conversations: *Acknowledging feelings and empathizing to build trust. Approaching conflicts with maturity through respectful dialogue. Embracing mistakes, supporting vulnerability, and exploring complexities for deeper understanding. Conversations vary in length from brief exchanges to extended discussions.*

Real conversations often unfold spontaneously, making them unpredictable and hard to structure in advance. Instead of imposing strict rules or demands, it's more effective to approach each conversation with self-awareness and an effort to find common ground. While you might not apply every suggestion offered here, being attentive to where conversations falter or listening to your daughter's feedback can inspire you to revisit these ideas and experiment with new approaches.

The goal isn't flawless conversations with zero challenges; it's about discovering better ways to listen and understand each other. What works one day may not work the next, so it's important to stay open to trying new approaches and ideas. As parents, it's our responsibility to lead by example, be creative, and find new ways to engage our girls in real conversations. By letting them know we're trying new things and learning as we go, we demonstrate humility and a willingness to learn, signaling how much we prioritize the relationship.

WIDEN YOUR PERSPECTIVE

I've worked with a lot of parents who firmly believe they know everything there is to know. They are convinced that their beliefs guarantee their child's safety and success, and they argue that any departure from their viewpoint poses risks and compromises their child's well-being. But in truth, any alternative perspective unsettles these parents, because it challenges their sense of safety.

Some people inherit a narrow view of life shaped by their parents' era, like the Great Depression, or family secrets and trauma. Their parents, molded by these challenges, teach them a specific way to cope. Even when these struggles change or fade, this narrow perspective stays, seen as the only path to stability. It cycles through generations, with other options seen as wrong or irresponsible.

There's always a rationale behind upholding this narrow perspective, whether it's the desire to maintain a certain reputation (*We raise our kids to be respectful*), to project or hold tight to a particular identity (*That's the way we do it in the South*), or simply a reluctance to face any questioning or uncertainty.

These are usually the parents who refuse to acknowledge when their daughter is angry or disconnected, and no matter what the challenge, they revert to the belief that one day they will be thanked and appreciated for upholding this specific approach to living. But in waiting for that one day, they miss out on every other day with their daughter. They miss the chance to share ordinary moments and grow closer as she gets older, ignoring how a lack of connection negatively affects her development.

Life is unpredictable and mysterious. While having a set of expectations and ideals to rely on can provide an inner sense of safety, they can't guarantee it. Clinging tightly to a specific viewpoint can inhibit our growth and understanding of others. Some girls may adhere to rules and expectations at home to maintain harmony, but others may struggle with it—not because they enjoy conflict, but because they recognize the need for a different, more inspiring, or creative approach to life. They are seeking to assert their individuality, trying to save themselves, or at least to be seen for who they are.

These girls, who opt for a nontraditional path, may eventually settle into a more conventional lifestyle—forming partnerships, raising children, and pursuing careers. But when they were young, they knew they had to find their own path. They needed to figure things out in a way that suited them, even if it eventually led them back to familiar outcomes. There are countless ways to navigate life, and each person has their own internal compass to guide them.

Our ability to broaden our perspective and make space for ideas beyond what we consider traditional keeps us connected to our girls as they navigate new terrain, reminding them that we are confident in who they are and what they can do.

Stability

As parents, if we refuse to listen, if we rely on simplistic answers, or if our responses are filled with certainty statements like, "Because I said so," it's a demonstration of a narrow, tightly controlled viewpoint and a lack of meaningful communication. This immediately blocks conversation and curiosity, and while the intention may be based in caring, the impact lands as an unwillingness to consider others.

A tightly controlled viewpoint is an attempt to find stability—*this is the answer, this is the decision, and that's the end of the conversation!* This has been sold to us as power or leadership, but for our girls, it translates as control and suppression. When there is a question or issue being debated, it's a great opportunity to listen with an open mind and practice objectivity. Yes, eventually decisions need to be made, but healthy leadership, which should ideally come from the parent, involves listening to each person and processing what's been said. In the end, the decision is still made, possibly the same decision the parent would have made without the input, but the communication and the connection are intact, resulting in mutual regard and respect.

Valuing a parenting approach with a strong sense of order and a strict adherence to rules understandably feels like stability. The world can feel overwhelming when there are so many choices, and stability and certainty are appealing. Personally, I've lost count of the number of parenting books I've read and the parents' groups I've led, all in the hope of finding definitive answers on how to sleep-train, stop certain behaviors, or determine what's best for my daughters.

We can find some guidance from data or other people's stories, but in the end our parenting experience is individual, unique, unpredictable. Even though my husband and I had three daughters, all raised in the same house, we still had to tailor our parenting to the distinctive needs of each girl, adapting to their personalities and life experiences.

We can view the world through a wider lens, understanding that there are numerous paths to a successful life, with multiple definitions of success. We can be open-minded enough to acknowledge that we are constantly learning, and that nothing is definitive or absolute. We need to embrace that things are always evolving, and real stability comes from our ability to accept and adapt.

What we can do to stabilize is take our traditional rules and reapply them in a new and compassionate way. Instead of having certainty about having the final word, we can have certainty that everyone deserves dignity. Instead of a strict adherence to outdated rules, we can have a strict adherence that everyone in the family feels seen. We can integrate the comfort of rules in a way that prioritizes human relationships over the rules themselves.

Messy

Girls tell me about the conversations with their parents where they end up yelling back and forth, calling each other names, slamming doors, or where they even avoid each other for days. These are heated arguments, filled with misunderstandings and unresolved conflicts, where everyone talks over each other, making it difficult to understand each other's perspectives. Emotions run high, leading to hurtful remarks and personal attacks, with topics shifting from one issue to another without resolution. Finding common ground seems impossible, and attempts at compromise are met with resistance or further conflict, leaving everyone feeling frustrated, drained, and disconnected.

This is not the kind of messy I would recommend, as it's inherently exhausting and, over time, harmful. Instead, I'm suggesting embracing a different definition of messy, where, during confusion and disagreement, we find a way to behave compassionately, even when everything feels emotionally charged or challenging. Though we may hold different opinions, we actively listen to each other without being overtly critical. We ask questions and remain open to expanding or changing our perspective. These conversations are messy because they are unpredictable and uncertain, but they're grounded in self-awareness and dignity, making sure that everyone feels seen and heard, even if a clear resolution isn't reached in the end.

In this way, "messy" is not seen as a negative word, but instead a creative word that invites us to embrace spontaneity and flexibility. Where we are free from rigid rules, where mistakes are expected, and we offer each other the grace to learn from them. It's helpful to associate messy with an open mind, or an ability to think freely. Our obsession with combatting messy by keeping our conversations "tidy" is an attempt to distract ourselves from uneasiness and reality, making it a coping tool to avoid what's uncomfortable.

Interacting with our daughters is not a one-way experience; we grow and change alongside them. Parenting is an art discovered through never-ending practice, where "messy" doesn't mean bad, but instead liberated and unexpected. The goal is the willingness to engage in the messy truth about life, to not hide from it by numbing out or running away through over-productivity and perfectionism. As parents, it's our job to support our girls in seeing and embracing it all, to view messy as an observance of reality rather than a shame to avoid.

Much of what our girls experience in the world isn't tidy at all, so buttoned-up conversations with absolute answers will inevitably fall flat. Contradictory opinions, generational differences, shifting emotions, and even the weather outside can all play a role in how a conversation unfolds. Our ability to normalize this messiness, rather avoid it, can make a difference in how our girls experience us.

For those of us who grew up in an authoritarian household, where parents or caregivers enforced a "my way or the highway" mentality, engaging in messy conversations can feel inherently incorrect, uncomfortable, or entirely foreign. *Authoritarian parenting* centers on parental obedience and control, emphasizing power and dominance, often neglecting the nurturing aspect of the parent-child relationship. Authoritarian parenting practices are still around, but less common, with research pointing to how they can lead to children having difficulties with socialization, decision-making, and their overall emotional well-being.

Permissive parents take the opposite approach, often showing minimal regard for rules and boundaries and sidestepping any conversations due to discomfort or distraction. A lax structure and unenforced expectations result in children feeling insecure in their unpredictable environment, leading to challenges with self-regulation and control. A parent dealing with addiction, abuse, or a mental health crisis may be considered an *uninvolved parent*, where the consistently uncertain environment leads to the child taking on the parenting role (the clinical word is *parentification*).

The most effective and evidence-based approach to raising children is considered *authoritative parenting*, where parents are not only supportive, but also attuned to their children's needs. Setting and upholding limits and expectations, with a strong focus on communication, values, and providing the reasoning behind rules, is central. It emphasizes the importance of building a relationship as the child grows.

Mistakes are expected, making it less about communicating perfectly, and more about being courageous enough to engage. Resilience is built through making mistakes and finding a way through them. This leads to trust and intimacy over time, allowing our girls to feel comfortable accepting and discussing their less-than-perfect lives, and parents who are willing to be less than perfect.

Understanding that life is indeed messy will always be the first obstacle. Metaphorically, there is duality—black/white, war/peace, good/bad—but in reality, every decision and discussion contain nuance. Life is subtle, less definitive, and we are constantly forced to wrestle with the paradox of opposing expectations: *You're perfect as you are, but keep improving; relationships can offer fulfillment and happiness, but relationships can never make you truly happy; be wise, but keep making mistakes; live a contemplative and thoughtful life, but know that too much thinking leads to neuroses.*

We are forced to live in the gray, often messy, space between, and to realize that's what it means to be human. People make a huge effort to exude a perfectly tidy external reality through having the right clothes, car, and house, but the over-effort is a distraction from the confusion going on inside. But it's in our best interest, as well as our daughters', to give confusion some room to be seen and understood—not to define it or believe we can solve it, but simply to discuss it and allow it to be.

There are beautiful and exhilarating moments inside messiness; there is growth and learning. And there is also discomfort and unpredictability that can leave us feeling vulnerable, or that we must be doing it wrong. *We aren't doing it wrong.* The messier a situation seems, the more opportunity we have to engage with complexity and widen our perspective.

People-Pleasing

I actively avoided messy conversations in my early life, with my default traits revolving around people-pleasing, allowing others to guide the conversation, and adapting to every scenario like a chameleon. It served me well in some ways, in that it kept me out of unnecessary drama, allowed me to be a good listener to those in need, and allowed me to navigate many different social groups. I was good at saying what people needed to hear and adjusting myself to fit their expectations.

But, as time went on, I recognized that this had significant limitations. I neglected my own needs because I never considered them or expressed them to others, and I was rarely acting in my integrity; instead, I was accommodating the people around me without considering myself. Surrendering to everyone else's needs made me feel like I was living a life that didn't belong to me, and it led to depression, anxiety, and underlying resentment.

I also recognized the cultural expectation for women to prioritize pleasing others and meeting everyone else's needs. Our societal conditioning emphasizes the role of women as caregivers, encouraging us to be agreeable and avoid causing disruptions. We're not-so-subtly encouraged to shrink ourselves, speak softly, and maintain a pleasant demeanor in public. When women express themselves too boldly, they are often labeled as domineering, overly dramatic, or aggressive. Even if they achieve remarkable success or assume leadership positions, they are frequently met with comments like, "There's just something about her that I don't like…"

For me, things changed when I became a mother to my first daughter and realized I could no longer remain silent and continue to appease everyone around me. I was now a grown woman, a wife, a therapist, and a mother, and if I didn't speak up for myself, I would not only drown in other people's expectations, I would also teach my daughter to do the same.

Without knowing how things would play out, I took a leap of faith and began asserting myself and expressing my needs. Sometimes, it felt like turning on a faucet too forcefully, where I came on too strong, struggling to regulate my emotions and find the right words to express myself effectively. Other times, I overly relied on someone else to initiate a difficult conversation by picking up on my body language or passive-aggressive attitude, and once the topic was open, I would share. With time, I learned to modulate and take more personal responsibility for what I wanted to say, but real conversations are always a work in progress.

My initial and most important conversations were with my husband, about how we could more equitably share household and childcare responsibilities and both pursue our careers, rather than falling into traditional gender roles where he continued to advance his career while I stepped back from mine. I also didn't want to be the only one focused on the day-to-day needs of our girls while he faced far fewer expectations as a father.

In heterosexual relationships, women often bear the brunt of invisible or cognitive labor—unseen and unpaid tasks like managing schedules and planning family activities, necessary for running a home and a family. As Eve Rodsky highlights in *Fair Play: A Game-Changing Solution for When You Have Too Much to Do*, society expects women to work as if they don't have children and raise children as if they don't work.

Research on housework and childcare tends to overlook this type of cognitive labor, and this is a significant oversight. Women not only perform more physical tasks at home, contributing to the gender pay gap and increased stress, but they also take on more of this mental load. Ignoring cognitive labor means we significantly underestimate the true extent of gender inequality and its impact on well-being.

Todd and I have hosted the *Zen Parenting Radio* podcast for nearly fourteen years, dedicating at least three or four episodes each year to the topic of cognitive labor. We continually discuss and redefine it as our girls grow older and their needs—and our tasks—evolve.

I also took the initiative to have honest conversations with my friends and family, expressing my true feelings about feeling disappointed, my political viewpoints, or simply sharing an opinion on a restaurant, rather than always saying, "Whatever you want!"

I started asking for help when needed and stopped pretending I was "fine" all the time. As my three daughters have grown up, I've made a conscious effort to confront the conversations that intimidate me the most. Hesitating to ask a question or share something significant is usually a sign that a conversation needs to happen.

Prioritizing a real, even messy, conversation allows us to prioritize ourselves, keeping our needs and desires at the forefront rather than succumbing to others' expectations of who we should be. By doing our best to engage, even when it feels uncomfortable, we create a culture of sharing ourselves and empowering our girls to do the same.

Instead of feeling intimidated by disagreements, our girls will recognize them as a normal part of life. Instead of being strangers to themselves, they will trust how they feel and learn how to articulate their thoughts and, even more important, actively listen to others.

This will help them navigate social media, work, and relationships genuinely, rather than conforming to societal expectations that encourage them to shrink or accommodate. It's like acquiring a lifelong superpower, equipping our girls to confront challenges with a sense of self and confidence.

SEE THEIR VIEWPOINT

As my daughter was getting ready for school, she shared how uncomfortable she was about her skin. Not only was it breaking out, but she had to stand up in class and share a poem that day, and everyone would be looking at her. She was also upset because she couldn't find socks to wear with her Converse shoes, and when I brought her a clean pair of socks, she was furious because she needed no-show socks, and the ones I'd brought would stick out and be noticeable.

She mentioned that she had to do group work during math, and her group consisted of one girl and three boys. She felt like they weren't getting anything done because the boys were messing around, but if she said anything to them, they said she was too serious and needed to relax. She also realized she had left part of the assignment at school, and when I suggested texting the girl in her group, she refused, saying she didn't want to appear needy or disorganized and preferred to deal with it herself.

Due to the pressure they feel, our girls are hyper-focused on themselves, believing that everyone else is equally fixated on their appearance, actions, words, or lack thereof. They harbor a deep fear of being seen as awkward or "awk," prompting them to conceal parts of their authentic selves, as if their true nature is too much for others to handle. It becomes instinctive for them to downplay their authenticity or emotions to fit into perceived social norms, and they become adept at pretending—diminishing their needs, passion, quirks, or intensity—to feel loved, or simply to be liked.

Their perspective incorporates a constant feeling of inadequacy, and they believe that others are scrutinizing them relentlessly. They hold a distorted self-image and believe that everyone they encounter is hyper-aware of, not only their appearance, but what they are thinking. If someone looks away, smiles, or passes them by without acknowledgment, they take it personally, assuming it's something they did wrong. While this experience can be true for all genders, it is particularly intense for our girls due to societal beauty standards and expectations of niceness, conformity, and the pressure to show up as responsible and likable.

Understanding this sensitivity is necessary when interacting with our girls because they closely observe and absorb our behavior, integrating it into their worldview. They are constantly assessing whether we will judge them, whether they can trust us, and whether they can share openly in our presence and be their authentic selves at home. This means we need to be aware of how we share our own perspective if we want them to feel seen and understood at home.

This is why it's vital to not only see their perspective, but also monitor our viewpoint. We need to question how we are perceiving what's happening in front of us—for instance, our ability to discern our daughters' body language and nonverbal cues. Paying close attention to signs such as crossed arms or frustrated glances provides valuable information for monitoring conversations when they veer off track. This is also a reminder to be thoughtful of our tone and body language, because that's what our girls really notice. They respond less to our words and more to the energy we bring to each conversation.

Understanding

Our girls don't just share about their own lives; they also share or discuss the lives of others in their world. It's a privilege to hear such personal information, and they trust that we can maintain a sense of maturity and kindness when they share. This means we need to be mindful and not use harsh criticism, judgment, gossip, or name-calling. Our job as adults is to find ways to communicate and not cause offense.

In some conversations, we may say the wrong thing, make mistakes, and then face resistance from our daughters, but their feedback helps us improve our communication and understand their perspective. We might get defensive initially when they tell us we're wrong or we hurt them, but listening and staying engaged is how we develop our relationship, and it's

A GUIDE FOR REAL CONVERSATIONS

how we practice and model how to communicate with others. As adults, it's our responsibility to learn how to avoid causing offense, rather than placing the burden on our daughters to not feel offended.

For those of us who grew up in families where listening to just one authority figure or adhering to a single belief system was the norm, this might be a new experience. We probably learned that any discomfort we felt was our fault or our misperception, and that negative comments from our parents were something we were expected to believe and accept.

As parents, we need to acknowledge when we secretly, or openly, believe there's only one right way to do things (our way), and when we're biased against people who look or live differently. We need to recognize when our strong beliefs are getting in the way of understanding our daughters' point of view, current experiences, or relationships.

To connect with this generation of girls—our daughters and their friends—we need to put ourselves in their shoes. We need to resist the idea that this generation is getting it wrong and past generations got everything right. It's typical to blame each new generation for being more difficult and naïve, and for disrupting all our cultural norms.

We may hold our own opinions about the past, believing that our experiences were special or correct. (They were special, and likely correct in their time!) But as time moves on, things change and evolve, and every generation looks and sounds different. The more we embrace the evolution of opinions and life choices, the greater the opportunity to see our similarities. Everyone, no matter their age, wants the same things: to express themselves, to be themselves, and to be deeply understood by those they care about.

One of the greatest challenges parents deal with is disentangling their deeply held beliefs from their identity. When we solely define ourselves by our opinions, shifting from them or considering something new feels like a threat to our integrity or sense of self.

As parents, if we understood that change is expected and it's our job to stay curious and keep learning, then encountering new information from younger generations might not feel like such a personal threat. We can adopt what researcher Adam Grant refers to as "confident humility": feeling self-assured, but also staying open to learning and growth—basically, finding a balance between assertiveness and humility.

The goal within a family is less about everyone adhering to the exact same beliefs in every aspect of life, and more about offering dignity and love to each person in the family. This may look like agreement on certain issues, and on others, disagreement with a willingness to listen and learn. I have worked with too many families that have broken down or apart due to political or religious differences, as well as prejudices when it comes to someone's sexuality or gender identification.

Parents who are unaware or unprepared for the experiences or personal disclosures their daughters share may react with anger, distance, or defensiveness, misinterpreting everything shared as deliberate attempts to hurt them. As our girls navigate their growth and identity, it's important to recognize that what they are sharing is about them, not us.

Our job as adults is to help, support, and give them space to express who they are, to make their own decisions and grow from their experiences. Denying them the right to have a viewpoint on the world or their own sense of self causes pain for all involved, and if it persists long enough, it unfortunately can become irreparable.

A GUIDE FOR REAL CONVERSATIONS

Individuality

Our girls' disclosures may indicate a transition to a new reality—they've been soccer players and now they're ready to move on. They are good students, but now they say they are struggling and want to be assessed for ADHD. You assumed they were straight, but they shared that they are gay. These revelations may feel difficult or uncomfortable because we didn't know or expect them, and we may need some time to process and reflect. The ultimate goal is to stay connected with our girls, prioritizing understanding over proving them wrong or rigidly sticking to the initial plan. As they evolve, so do our approaches.

When girls feel seen, heard, and supported in their identities, they are more likely to trust themselves and navigate the world with confidence. By affirming and celebrating who they are, we create a supportive environment where they can feel safe to move toward their fullest potential.

This generation of young women is not a monolith, but most of the girls I talk to share a similar perspective about being true to themselves and expressing their individuality. They also question traditional stereotypes and societal norms, and prefer to express themselves in ways that reflect who they truly are. They view themselves as catalysts for change, not necessarily by choice, but by need—so they engage in, or at least have a lot of knowledge about, social movements that address issues like equality, racial and social justice, common-sense gun laws, and climate change.

They are immersed in their online world, using technology to express themselves and make connections. They openly discuss mental health, and they actively seek therapeutic help while also working to destigmatize it. They are deeply worried about their future, feeling incredibly anxious about legislation that has already impacted their reproductive rights and autonomy over their bodies. Many young girls are ambivalent about having children of their own, believing that it's irresponsible given the current global challenges. They see their own lives as totally different from ours, and thinking we can force them into our way of thinking ignores the culture they live in and the challenges they face.

Every generation needs supportive parents and wisdom from their elders, so we, of course, can share insights and our experiences, but we need to adopt a more flexible approach with less rigid insistence that our view is the only right view. Girls tell me how frustrating it is to feel dismissed by their parents, especially when they hear variations of statements like, "You don't know stress or responsibility; you're just a kid without a job." This overlooks the reality that these young women are facing, how they are exposed to the complexities of the world—disinformation, active shooter drills—while witnessing international violence through their devices. Denying their struggles undermines their experiences and prevents them from seeing us as a safe place to share.

We may deny or discredit our girls' experiences because our viewpoints were disregarded when we were young. Instead of learning to value our own opinions, we were forced to embrace the opinions of our authority figures. Now, as parents in a position of authority, we believe it's our turn to be heard and valued. It's true, we have accumulated a lifetime of experiences and wisdom to share, but there's a distinction between sharing and forcing. Sharing is typically requested and appreciated, while forcing will inevitably be met with defense and rejection.

Respecting our girls' individuality means allowing them to confidently express their perspectives in every aspect of their lives. If we neglect to listen, and instead impose our own views or persistently insist that they are wrong, it's a lot more probable that our daughters will adopt similar behavior in their future relationships. This typically unfolds in one of two ways: either they learn to force their opinions on others, or they learn to let others force opinions onto them.

A GUIDE FOR REAL CONVERSATIONS

ENCOURAGE CRITICAL THINKING

Our daughters, and society as a whole, are in dire need of critical thinking skills. We're dealing with a serious problem of polarization and a decline in trust in facts and science, and many people are relying on social media and less reliable sources for information. Encouraging our daughters to analyze information objectively and engage in discussions with various, even contradictory, perspectives at home increases the likelihood that they will develop a critical mindset. Viewing things as only good or bad, or as black or white, makes it difficult for them to understand the complexity in every situation.

We can start by engaging with smaller things, like when our girls say, "The whole school is talking about me," or "I'm a failure at everything." We know this is exaggerating or catastrophizing, but we can lead with curiosity by asking them why they think this, or what happened that made them feel this way. We can ask them if they've ever felt this way before, or if they think other people ever feel this way. We can do our best to get them to consider many different perspectives without telling them what to think.

Immediately pushing back or denying what they feel only puts them in a defensive position, and most likely ends the conversation. But being curious and allowing them to share gives them an opportunity to untangle it on their own. Then they can come to recognize that the whole school is not talking about them, but they do feel vulnerable, or that they aren't a failure at everything, but they are feeling uneasy about some of their abilities.

We can also explore objectivity through events in the news, or pop culture, from various angles. Instead of rushing to judgment about who is good or bad, right or wrong, we can discuss issues from many different angles. When a celebrity faces criticism for something they said, we can discuss what happened, different ways to address it, the media's role and how it's being reported, social media's response and judgment, and how the whole thing is a complex debate rather than clear-cut answers. Conversations like these allow our girls to see a bigger picture and notice many different viewpoints that can help them formulate their own.

In today's world, facts are easily questioned or distorted, so it's important for us to help our girls distinguish between facts and opinions. We can guide them by identifying shows and newspapers that are strictly opinion-based versus resources with journalistic integrity. We can also discuss what bias looks like and the value of fact-checking, and how some people just lie to win arguments.

Objectivity is what they need to actively participate in meaningful class discussions, workplace issues, and even their friendships and romantic relationships. It allows them to see things clearly from many different perspectives, offering them the ability to step back and consider all the facts alongside their feelings. It's about seeing things in a multidimensional way, not just through the lens of their most vulnerable or highly stressed selves.

Misogyny & Culture

In the social work classes I teach, we explore the impact of misogyny, with students openly sharing their encounters with sexism and its effects. According to Kate Manne in *Down Girl: The Logic of Misogyny*, sexism justifies patriarchal social orders, while misogyny enforces the norms that uphold them. For example, in a high-level college classroom, a teacher might call on young men more frequently than young women, assuming male students are more capable (sexism). And when a female student confidently speaks up, she may face interruptions, dismissals, or questioning, while similar behavior from male students is encouraged and praised (misogyny).

Misogyny is typically attributed to men, but women can also internalize and perpetuate oppressive beliefs due to their upbringing and cultural conditioning. These ideas can lead to their own self-criticism, judgment of others, and behaviors aimed at conforming to societal norms to avoid any negative consequences. Some women, consciously or unconsciously, believe aligning with men will offer them safety.

In class we also discuss misogynoir, which is a specific type of misogyny rooted in racism. Coined by feminist scholar, writer, and activist Moya Bailey in 2010, the term blends "misogyny" with the French word for black, "noir." My Black, female students share their experiences around getting viewed as older than they are, more mature, and more sexually advanced than white girls, which contributes to the disbelief or dismissal of allegations involving the sexual abuse of Black girls and teens. Black girls and women are frequently stereotyped as sassy, angry, strong, or overly sexual, which not only limits and oppresses them, but also restricts their ability to express their individuality.

Misogynoir shows up in a variety of ways, such as doctors believing Black women have a higher pain threshold, which results in them receiving different treatment, and maternal mortality rates for Black women in the United States being three times higher than those for white women. Then, when Black women advocate for themselves and seek appropriate treatment, they are often perceived as threatening or angry.

Styles that are considered unacceptable on Black girls are often celebrated on white girls, where Black women may face criticism in school or professional settings for natural hairstyles like afros or braids, while these same styles are trendy on white women. Similarly, in sports, outfits worn by Black athletes, such as Serena Williams' scrutinized catsuit at the 2018 French Open, can spark bans or controversy, contrasting with the praise received by white athletes for similar attire.

The Latina girls in my classroom share the impact of machismo or hypermasculinity in their culture and how it affects their home environments. Machismo reinforces male dominance over women and coexists with Marianismo, which defines women as homemakers, mothers, and caretakers of the family. Passed down through generations in Latin culture, machismo creates an environment where men are taught to exert control and to believe they must be stronger than and superior to women.

Machismo defines traditional gender roles, where women are assigned household and familial duties while men focus on providing income and labor. A lot of my students have had to bring their siblings or cousins with them to our classroom because they are expected to care for them during the day. Additionally, these girls often lack adequate support to continue their education because they are needed at home for childcare, managing household responsibilities, or serving as translators.

The girls share that their greatest struggles have been to gain their fathers' support, or to support their mothers, whom they perceive as lacking agency. Especially girls who are firstborns feel pressure to be obedient and prioritize their home life and future family over their college education. These expectations from a young age limit their opportunities, and often discourage them from pursuing careers, particularly in male-dominated spaces.

A quick note about preferred language regarding race and ethnicity: Race categorizes people based on physical characteristics, while ethnicity relates to cultural identity, including customs, history, language, and religion. Race is often seen as inherited, while ethnicity is learned cultural identification. Because each girl has her own story, I've learned to ask about their preferences, a practice that also applies to gender and sexuality (see LGBTQ+ section on page 100).

In this chapter, I use the language my students have requested while recognizing the variations in how people choose to identify. BIPOC (Black, Indigenous, and People of Color) is commonly used to center the experiences of Black and Indigenous groups. When speaking with Black girls in my class, most prefer simply "Black." Latina girls currently prefer "Latina" (or "Latino" when referring to their families). Around five years ago, "Latinx" was preferred, so I used that. I follow their lead as preferences evolve. I share this because girls have strong feelings about the language used to identify them, providing another opportunity to be curious and ask.

Across many cultures and traditions, expectations rooted in misogyny persist, and our girls feel these challenges early on as they navigate the balance between family expectations and their own modern aspirations. Without discussions and reflection, they easily internalize cultural norms as just facts, rather than recognizing them as products of cultural conditioning.

We can set an example of feminism in our family relationships and marriage, choose diverse books, toys, and movies, and prioritize intelligence and resilience over appearance. But these steps are only the beginning. We need to engage our girls in conversations about the world and affirm what they themselves are experiencing and observing.

It's important to discuss the reality that plenty of people and groups view women as inferior, and ignoring or pretending otherwise creates a false reality. While we can be hopeful about progress and discuss and advocate for positive changes, it's equally important to acknowledge the existence of barriers and confront the fact that bigotry persists. Many parents, especially fathers I've spoken to, often avoid these conversations, hoping to personally reassure their daughters of their worth and shield them from societal biases. But our daughters can't escape what they witness and hear. Addressing these issues doesn't reinforce stereotypes; it helps dismantle them.

I listen every week to the *Armchair Expert* podcast, hosted by Dax Shepard and Monica Padman. Within their network, they feature a variety of podcasts, including one called *Synced*, where Monica and author Liz Plank engage in weekly conversations. Recently, Monica shared that a male friend of hers listens to all the podcasts on their network except *Synced*, because it features two women and he felt it didn't pertain to him.

This belief is pervasive: that men can only relate to what other men say and struggle to connect with topics discussed among women about life and their experiences. It's not just about listening to women's stories; it's also about men being able to see themselves or find resonance in women's stories. Throughout history, women have had to see themselves through men—whether through historical figures, literary characters, or movie heroes. Representation is important and is needed more than ever, but women have long been expected to find themselves through the male experience.

I did my own research and asked all the men I know which podcasts they listen to—specifically, if they listen to any podcasts where two or more women are in conversation without any men. Not one man said he did. This example highlights how deeply ingrained it is to perceive men's viewpoints as the default, and women's viewpoints as niche. This is evident in terms like "chick flicks" for certain movies, or separate "women's books" sections in bookstores, while other movies and books with male authors or leads are simply movies and books.

A GUIDE FOR REAL CONVERSATIONS

Alison Bechdel—a cartoonist who achieved critical and commercial success with her graphic memoir *Fun Home*, which was adapted into a musical that won a Tony Award—introduced a significant new standard in media critique with the Bechdel Test. To pass, a film or TV episode must meet three criteria:

1. It must include at least two women.
2. These women must have a conversation with each other.
3. The conversation should be about something other than a man.

There's sometimes an additional requirement that these female characters are named and play a meaningful role in the plot, rather than being background figures. As of April 2024, the website BechdelTest.com assessed about 9,800 films and found that only 57 percent of these films passed all three of the test's requirements, with 10 percent failing one requirement, 22 percent failing two, and 11 percent failing all three.

Acknowledging and naming these issues validates what our daughters experience. It ensures that everyday slights or major injustices are understood as failures of the system, not reflections on themselves. These often-overlooked societal norms can help us recognize the disparities in our experiences.

During my early twenties, when I lived in Chicago, a man in the neighboring house would flash me—literally take down his pants in front of the window—as I walked past his place. When I told my three roommates, they shared that he had done the same to them. One day, while mentioning yet another flashing incident to one of my roommates' boyfriends who happened to be visiting, he was visibly shocked and asked why we hadn't called the police. It was challenging to convey to him all the things we had experienced—catcalls from men who followed us home, men who exposed themselves to us on the L train and bus, truck drivers who honked and tailed us as we drove to work, men who walked by us on the sidewalk and told us to pay attention to them, or that we should be smiling. These experiences, sadly very common for young women, can numb us to their seriousness.

When I share these stories with my daughters, they're also shocked by some of the things my friends and I experienced, but plenty of similar stories exist in their generation: sexist, violent, and misogynistic social media posts and trolling comments; classroom remarks about girls that are met with laughter instead of reprimand; incidents of revenge porn that are shared; and girls being ostracized for standing up for others or challenging sexist remarks.

Our girls need to feel safe sharing their experiences with us without fear of blame, knowing that behavior like this—whether online or in person—is unacceptable. They should feel comfortable asking us difficult questions, confident that we can listen and process what they are saying. Above all, our girls should never feel guilty or blame themselves if they find themselves targeted.

Cults and High-Control Groups

When our girls seek connections with others, the internet and its many platforms open a world of possibilities to find new friends and communities worldwide. But it also means they may encounter people or groups who might not have their best intentions at heart.

Our daughters can easily find themselves stuck in echo chambers, where they're bombarded with information that reinforces only one perspective. This can lead to confirmation bias, where they seek out information that already aligns with their existing beliefs and ignoring anything that doesn't. Social media algorithms make this issue much worse, leading

A GUIDE FOR REAL CONVERSATIONS

to endless scrolling that inevitably shapes our daughters' perceptions of the world and influences their overall judgment.

Right now, we are in the "golden age" of cults because there's a wealth of books and documentaries uncovering various cults and how they indoctrinate people. They highlight how digital technology influences the spread of information, and there is a focus on the importance of promoting critical thinking to guard against being easily influenced.

The groups that need to be avoided are considered high-control groups, characterized by strict regulation of behavior, beliefs, and interactions, with hierarchies and rigid rules. They exert their influence through social pressure, conformity, and obedience to authority figures. Cults are a subset of high-control groups that use extreme tactics, such as isolation, indoctrination, and exploitation of members.

Cults usually feature a charismatic and narcissistic leader who demands loyalty, and this leader presents a worldview that discourages questioning, dividing followers into an in-group and an out-group based on their acceptance or rejection of this worldview. Good and evil are defined according to what serves the group's interests, and followers are urged to abandon their critical thinking abilities.

Conspiracy theories and cults often go hand in hand, even though they're not identical. Aspiring cult leaders tend to adopt or create conspiracy theories to find followers who share their beliefs. Those who already acknowledge society's flaws are drawn to cult leaders because they want a new perspective to challenge the flawed status quo, which is what these leaders offer.

Many parents are unaware that their daughters could be vulnerable to high-control groups or cults, and sometimes it's the parents themselves who are involved in these groups, with their children attempting to awaken them to the group's influence. These groups are everywhere and often fly under the radar. They can show up in religion, politics, fitness groups, and even in toxic one-on-one relationships where someone is manipulative and using abusive, cult-like tactics.

We can openly discuss with our daughters how to recognize warning signs and red flags indicating they may be targeted. These tactics may include overwhelming affection (love bombing), gaslighting (making them doubt their own reality), isolation from others, and inducing feelings of guilt or shame.

Love bombing is when someone excessively showers another with affection, attention, compliments, and gifts at the start of a relationship to speed up the development of feelings of deep love and acceptance. The love bomber might come off as charming and perfect, making you feel deeply connected and fortunate. But their real goal is to gain power over you, and once they feel like they've got your trust and emotional dependence, they start controlling and manipulating.

Gaslighting is used to make someone doubt their own perceptions, memories, and sanity. The term comes from the play and movie *Gaslight*, where a husband makes his wife believe she's going insane by dimming the gaslights in their home and then denying it when she notices. These days, "gaslighting" is often thrown around when someone simply has a different opinion or questions what we believe, but that's just normal disagreement. Real gaslighting involves denying events or experiences, minimizing the person's feelings or concerns, blaming the victim, and using repetition or misdirection to confuse them. The goal of gaslighting is to break down someone's confidence and sense of reality, making them easier to control and less likely to trust themselves.

Isolation is used to control by disconnecting people from their friends, family, and other support networks. This can involve controlling access to communication, like the phone or social media, monitoring interactions with others, and discouraging or prohibiting socializing with anyone else. The objective is to create dependence and make it difficult to ask for help or leave the situation easily.

Guilt and shame are used to make people feel bad about themselves and undermine their confidence, leading them to believe there's something inherently wrong with who they are. They're often made to feel ashamed of normal flaws or mistakes, as if perfection is expected. In high-control groups or cults, people might be guilt-tripped into revealing personal information, which is then used to shame or blackmail them.

It's much easier to address these topics early on, rather than trying to explain them when our girls are already becoming involved with someone or a group that insists on conformity. We don't have to scare them or use fear tactics; instead, we can help them develop their own critical thinking skills and remind them of the importance of their own thoughts and decision-making. If this becomes a value in our home, where everyone is heard and has a right to their opinion, it makes them less susceptible to being drawn into situations where they're expected to abandon their beliefs and adhere to someone else's fear-based worldview.

A daughter getting good grades, who is told she's loved, or who has found some success through sports or clubs, is not necessarily immune to being drawn into harmful situations, and conversations about recognizing red flags are still necessary. People who believe they would never be pulled into a cult are often the most susceptible. I've worked with outwardly successful girls who have still been drawn into harmful relationships or social circles, or high-control religions or groups. Plus, so many older high school girls, and certainly a significant portion of my college students, have shared with me their experiences of being in at least one emotionally or physically abusive relationship.

Critical thinking skills are crucial for spotting and deflecting manipulation tactics used by harmful people, and they're also valuable for assessing relationships and friendships. While we don't want our girls to become overly critical, we can encourage them to be skeptical of easy fixes for life's most complex problems.

Manipulative individuals often offer simple answers to complex questions, promising clarity in a confusing world. Statements such as "Join our group, and you'll never be alone," "Follow me, I'm the only one who can keep you safe," or "Date me, and you'll always be loved," can be tempting, especially for girls who feel isolated or unsure of themselves.

Belonging & Certainty

I've worked with a lot of women and girls who've been abused, women who've gotten wrapped up in groups like QAnon and spiritual wellness circles, and I've had my own experiences with cult-like situations and emotionally abusive relationships. I never joined a well-known cult, but I have walked several cult-like paths. As a yoga teacher and a member of the wellness industry, I have witnessed scandals and the downfall of teachers and thought leaders, and I have been hurt by wellness "experts" who claimed to have elevated spirituality or a heightened ability to help people.

I have had teachers who initially helped me and then later hurt me, leading to cognitive dissonance about what is considered healthy and what is considered toxic. I have watched people I once trusted be corrupted by fame, power, money, or sex, leaving their followers to grapple with hypocrisy and damage.

I have also worked with teachers who taught me to live a more self-aware and connected life. I have known authors, therapists, and yoga practitioners who showed up genuinely and demonstrated a compassionate way of living. These people live with humility and act humanely, walking the walk of what they teach. Their approach doesn't rely on easy solutions or positioning themselves as the sole authorities. Instead, they encourage others to challenge perspectives, and refrain from oversimplifying complex issues.

That's why I'm kind of obsessed with studying cults and extremist groups, because I found myself in several coercive groups that bordered on high-control, and I came pretty damn close to being sucked into some bad situations. I understand the appeal of belonging and the certainty that these groups offer. They make you feel understood, special, and even superior to others. They create a sense that you perceive the world clearly while others do not, or that you have access to the answers, giving you an advantage over everyone else. I also know that people who join these communities are often well-meaning seekers, eager to find ways to contribute positively and relieve their anxiety about the world.

A dogma, cause, or belief that offers purpose and certainty is hard to resist. These groups, teachers, and sometimes even abusive partners, create initial highs that make us feel alive, seen, and valued, and we do everything we can to hold on to or recreate these experiences, even when we see red flags everywhere. I found myself seeking these spiritual and psychological highs for a lot of my adult life. I gained some valuable insights, but I also experienced emotional and spiritual exploitation. There are always elements of truth in what is offered, but without critical thinking, we can easily overlook the reality and our own safety.

My experience in the world of yoga teacher training is one of many examples. At first, my yoga training was about the basics, but it gradually morphed into a quest for the perfect yoga attire and the top-tier mat, all while feeling pressured to achieve the highest level of accreditation. Most of the time and money I invested in accreditation was nullified by allegations against the leader of the yoga style I was studying. The allegations included a sex scandal, financial mismanagement, and coercion and manipulation of students. Even within the realm of yoga, there exists a cult of personality, where some teachers exploit their "spirituality" for financial gain and power.

I've also had yoga teachers who excelled at their practice, on and off the mat, and helped me develop a better understanding of the meaning of integrity. They never forced a belief system or demanded obedience; they promoted freedom of thought and allowed me to learn at my own pace. Since both experiences are real, it became, and remains, my responsibility to discern how I view and experience yoga. Right now, I no longer teach, but I still take classes. I also practice yoga on my front porch, in sweatpants, on a ten-dollar mat, while listening to a podcast.

Discernment & Humility

There is a kind of certainty that makes sense. If we touch a hot stove and learn that it burns, we stop touching the stove. But applying the same rules and logic to more complex situations doesn't work. Having a relationship that breaks our heart doesn't mean we should stop having relationships, and being fired from a job doesn't mean we don't have anything to offer the world. Great learning can come from challenging situations. If we are willing, they have the power to evolve our thinking and develop our resilience.

But if we lack curiosity or a desire to learn, challenging situations can push us into a place of fear, where certainty is needed and unpredictability cannot be tolerated. Instead of humility, there is only digging in and doubling down, which inevitably becomes extreme or fanatical. There is a reliance on binary thinking where any disagreement becomes a threat, so you are either with me and good, or against me and bad.

A GUIDE FOR REAL CONVERSATIONS

Binary thinking relies on either/or scenarios, even though most situations are more nuanced, involving both/and perspectives. Overcoming binary thinking can be challenging because it boosts our egos and creates a clear "us versus them" mentality. We feel secure when surrounded by like-minded people and threatened when our beliefs are challenged. Binary thinking only serves to create division, and we need to have more nuanced discussions, especially in our families, to develop a deeper understanding of complex issues.

You might recognize yourself or others here, in situations involving religion, politics, or even marriage and parenting. This doesn't mean that we should abandon religion, politics, or family altogether; it just suggests that some people and organizations have been hijacked and damaged by a desire for power or certainty. This is why it's important to practice discernment—to question and look rationally at our feelings and needs, and to lean on the support of those we love and trust the most.

By adopting a more self-aware and inquisitive approach to life, we can reduce our interactions with self-serving individuals and institutions. And if it's family members or loved ones who insist on a certain way of thinking, it might allow us an opportunity to communicate more effectively, with clear boundaries and awareness.

While we can make attempts to listen and understand different perspectives, we do not need to engage with people or groups that promote hate, violence, or dehumanization. And we can also recognize the BITE model, developed by Steven Hassan, which describes specific methods cults use to recruit and maintain control over people by manipulating behavior, information, thought, and emotions (BITE). These are significant red flags that may necessitate additional or professional support and guidance.

Discernment lives at the heart of our ability to take care of ourselves, to notice our emotions and engage with our critical thinking. There is comfort in believing that we have a right answer to every question, but there are few things that are this cut-and-dried, and several things are always true at once. We need to recognize and talk with our girls about paradoxical challenges, like, *You can give your all and still need to back out. You can be resilient and still need a break. You can be independent and still need others.*

Humility, or even confusion, are not weaknesses or indicators of a lack of confidence. They represent the ultimate form of confidence—a willingness to question ourselves and stay open to new information. The opposite of humility is recognizing flaws only in other people's ideas or opinions, while ignoring our own. This type of arrogance makes for a challenging partner, parent, or leader.

So many girls I talk to struggle to know for sure or make the one right choice, when there is no such thing. There are only different choices depending on the situation, experience, or moment. There are choices that others will want you to make, and then there is the choice you make, based on your specific set of circumstances, right now, today.

People like to believe that things are black and white because they desperately want the security and want so badly to be right, but they eventually realize—hopefully—that life exists in the gray areas and solace is found somewhere in the middle. Seeing things from many different angles is a telltale sign that we are becoming wise.

I've opened up to my daughters about my past experiences with cultish situations, and they still remember individuals and aspects from those periods, when I was obsessed with the latest book, teacher, or self-improvement workshop. I've encouraged them to watch a few documentaries about high-control groups and cults so they recognize how similar tactics are used to coerce and abuse people, and how to pay attention to red flags so they can be spotted early on.

At the same time, I am still a yogi, the founder of an annual parenting conference, and the host of a podcast where we discuss personal growth. I don't think we need to discard the good with the bad. We just need to recognize when we are out of our integrity or when we are feeling trapped, obligated, or isolated from others.

Our girls will inevitably have to learn some of these lessons through their own experiences, but we can proactively discuss these things with them and provide support as they navigate what feels right versus what feels obligatory and restrictive.

It's an ongoing conversation to help our girls navigate the delicate balance between trust and skepticism. While there are many positive influences in the world, there are also plenty of negative ones, and our goal is to empower them to develop and trust their own intuition.

Ideally, we've created a relationship and communication style where they feel comfortable coming to us when they're confused, without fearing shame or judgment. By sharing our belief in them and our willingness to listen, we increase the likelihood that our daughters will depend on themselves and their instincts.

ELIMINATE THESE PHRASES

After listening to my clients and students repeatedly recount the most common and cliché things their parents have said to them, I've narrowed it down to these six. There are variations, but these capture the essence and set the stage for damaging conversations.

Saying these things to our girls immediately creates a disconnection, showing our defensiveness and prompting our daughters to respond defensively as well. These tend to be default responses when we're emotionally drained, overwhelmed, or unsure of what to do or say next.

They are also obvious deflections when we feel afraid, vulnerable, or pressured to have all the answers. Many of us likely heard similar phrases while growing up, and we know how much they hurt and derail a conversation. But because they're familiar, they can easily slip out, becoming throwaway remarks that we later regret.

You're Too Sensitive

Telling our daughters they are "too sensitive" hurts because it brushes off their feelings as if they are unimportant or an overreaction. It implies that there's something inherently wrong with feeling deeply, reinforcing the idea that sensitivity is a weakness rather than a strength.

When we tell our girls that their feelings are a problem, it leaves them feeling inadequate and ashamed, as if their emotions aren't worthy of being acknowledged. Labeling them as "too sensitive" makes them question themselves, creating a situation where they hide what they feel and have difficulty asking for help when they need it most. Instead of offering support and guidance in navigating their emotions, this phrase ends up undermining their emotional well-being.

You're Being Dramatic

Similar to saying "you're too sensitive," telling our daughters they're being dramatic dismisses their feelings and, as they tell me, makes them feel embarrassed. It leaves them thinking their feelings don't count, or like they're blowing things out of proportion. Over time, this leads to a lack of trust in their own feelings or an inability to discern what truly bothers them, questioning whether they are overreacting or genuinely have something important to share. Telling them they're "being dramatic" also reinforces harmful stereotypes about girls, portraying them as overly emotional or irrational.

When we label our girls "drama queens," it's often a strategy to sidestep our own feelings or discomfort. Dismissing our girls' emotions as exaggerated shields us from confronting our own feelings, allowing us to feel justified in becoming annoyed with theirs. If we were taught, or believe, that emotions should be stifled or suppressed, it can make us feel uncomfortable, or even angry, when our daughters get to express theirs.

If our girls' reactions do appear exaggerated or overblown, it's often because they feel they need to overreact to be heard and get what they need. If their emotions have been disregarded in the past, they may feel they need to amplify them to gain attention. But if we consistently create an environment of understanding and acceptance toward feelings over time, our girls will be able to express themselves more genuinely, and the need to exaggerate will become less pressing.

I Told You So

When we offer advice and our girls don't take it, we so badly want validation that our advice was correct, and that, if only they had listened to us, they would be okay. This is a tough one for most parents. It goes without saying that we do know more than our girls—we have had more life experience to draw from, and we can see the world through an adult lens. We learned a lot of what we know through trial and error, and that's where our girls are right now. They are trying and failing, figuring things out along the way. Our desire for recognition, suggesting they should have listened to us, becomes self-serving and unsupportive. It stems from our need to feel valued and acknowledged by our daughters.

If we offer advice but they don't follow it, and then they have difficulties, responding with compassion and understanding is how we stay in the loop of communication. It can require effort on our part to acknowledge our own frustration and realize that "winning" the conversation doesn't need to be the ultimate goal. Responding with "I told you so" doesn't inspire their learning; it only leaves them annoyed at us, and usually ashamed.

Leading with compassion offers our daughters the opportunity to see for themselves that our advice held value. When we approach with humility and vulnerability, it usually invites a similar response. As parents, we hold the role of leaders, responsible for setting the tone for mature conversations. It's important to steer clear of righteousness or the need to win.

What's Wrong with You?

When someone you trust or rely on asks, "What's wrong with you?" it leads to painful questioning and self-doubt. Girls already feel as if something is wrong with them, so hearing this from someone they love feels scary. Girls have confided in me about hearing variations of this phrase, and they carry a distinct memory of when they heard it, how they felt, and the enduring memory of its impact. Limited by their own lack of life experience, they internalize this message as fact, leading to damaging thoughts such as "I'm not good enough" or "I'm a bad person."

If our daughter is behaving out of character or seeking attention, it's better to approach her with questions like, "Did something happen?" or "You don't seem like yourself, can I help?" This subtle shift from judgment to care acknowledges that there may be a story or underlying reasons for her behavior. It shows we're ready to listen without judging, creating a safe space to share. It also proves we're paying attention and are always here to help when she needs us.

You Always or You Never

I like to annoy my college students by quoting Wendell Johnson's wise words: "Always and never are two words you should always remember never to use." They roll their eyes, but it begins a valuable conversation about how these words are absolutes, painting things in black and white with no middle ground. Using "always" and "never" in a relational conversation leads to unnecessary drama and misunderstandings.

Using phrases like, "You always do that!" or "You're never going to get that done!" blows things out of proportion, making our daughters focus on every instance when they did or didn't do something, rather than focusing on the topic at hand.

Exaggeration happens when we want to get a big emotional reaction, especially if we feel like our message isn't getting through. We exaggerate our feelings, or the situation, because we believe it's the only way to emphasize the importance of what we're trying to say. But when we go overboard with dramatic gestures or words, we can lose sight of the real point we're trying to get across. It's better to keep things calm and straightforward instead of resorting to over-the-top tactics that can get in the way of what we are trying to convey.

I Don't Believe You

Saying "I don't believe you" is a deep wound for our girls, particularly given the stereotyping ingrained in our society about girls being dramatic or untrustworthy. From a young age, girls absorb messages that cast doubt on their thoughts and feelings, facing societal pressures that minimize their emotions and experiences. Many girls and women have experienced having their voices dismissed or silenced, whether at home or in professional settings, and internalize these doubts, which gradually erode their self-confidence.

Men's stories, opinions, memories, and emotions (especially anger) carry more weight in our culture, making women seem less credible, untrustworthy, and sometimes literally unbelievable. The message is clear in news, social media, and private conversations: *men matter a lot, women matter less.*

I've worked with girls who confided in their parents about being molested by a family member, only to face questioning or disbelief. Some parents, even if they do believe their daughters, choose to keep things quiet to avoid any disruption to the family. I've also worked with girls who bravely shared their rape experiences with their university or police, only to be questioned about their own role or told that nothing can be done.

My friend Jenny Zabrocki, MSW, a sexual assault counselor, has observed an encouraging trend: there's an increased likelihood of girls and women who report sexual assault being believed. The services that are provided to them after reporting focus on restoring their sense of agency, acknowledging the power that was taken from them during the assault. As a result, survivors feel empowered to make decisions regarding their care, such as whether to undergo a rape kit examination and who they want present during their intake and reporting process.

Still, Jenny has also noticed a reluctance among survivors and their families to pursue justice after reporting. This reluctance usually stems from a fear of causing trouble or making the abuser's life more difficult. Parents may also inadvertently contribute to this dynamic by focusing on what the girl did or didn't do, reinforcing an "I told you so" mentality. This blame-shifting leads survivors to feel partially responsible for the assault.

Jenny also points out how cultural differences influence the response to sexual assault. In Hispanic families, there's often a preference to keep such matters private or handle them internally. Similarly, in Black families, there's often less trust in the justice system, resulting in fewer reports of sexual assault and a reluctance to pursue justice. Mistrust and victim-blaming dynamics continue to be an issue, with greater emphasis placed on scrutinizing the survivor's actions than on addressing the perpetrator's behavior.

We've seen high-profile court cases where women were forced to recount the details of sexual assault or harassment, as seen in Anita Hill's case during the Clarence Thomas hearings. Similarly, Dr. Christine Blasey Ford shared her story of sexual assault during Brett Kavanaugh's Supreme Court confirmation process. Despite knowing their stories might not have the power to sway the outcome, women everywhere rallied around them, understanding and sharing similar experiences. They recognized the courage and sacrifices involved, and wanted these women to know they weren't alone.

Victims of abuse and harassment often face pressure to recall every detail of their experience and are even accused of lying for their own benefit they can't remember certain details. But there's a lack of information about how trauma affects memory. Traumatic experiences can disrupt both the formation and retrieval of memories, resulting in fragmented recollections, intrusive flashbacks, and distortions. While some memories may be quite vivid due to heightened emotions during the negative experience, survivors may find it difficult to remember less significant details because of the way trauma affects memory.

RESTORING OUR GIRLS

Consider 9/11: You likely recall where you were when you heard, and maybe you have some really specific details about the moment—your clothes, what the room smelled like, who was there. But if asked about your lunch that day, the commute home, or everybody you talked to on the phone that night, those details will be hazy and most likely impossible to recall. This selective memory doesn't invalidate your experience; it's a product of trauma's impact on memory. Understanding this is crucial if, as a culture, we want to be more trauma-informed.

I've yet to encounter a girl or woman who wants to alter and disrupt her life after an attack—or "seek attention or fame"—by reporting a false accusation. According to the National Violence Resource Center, over 63 percent of assaults aren't even reported, and for those that are, only somewhere between 2 and 7 percent are considered false reports.

Regardless, pursuing justice takes a toll, causing pain and upheaval to the survivor that can stretch on for years, disrupting every aspect of their life and their mental and physical well-being. If you want insight into the survivor's journey, I recommend reading Chantal Miller's powerful memoir, *Know My Name*. In her book, she shares the trauma, pain, and resilience of being a survivor, while also challenging societal attitudes toward sexual violence and advocating for justice and healing.

Telling our daughters "I don't believe you" is not always about violence or trauma; it can happen over simple matters, like when they are sharing their feelings, explaining their actions, or sharing whether or not they've finished a school assignment. Some parents might even escalate to calling their daughters liars, due to feeling frustrated or losing control of a situation.

Our daughters might lie to avoid disappointing us or losing privileges, or to protect their friends. Sometimes, the lie ends up digging them into a hole that's tough to climb out of—a very typical teen experience that we may all be able to relate to.

We want to trust them, and catching them in a lie triggers our anger, making us reactive and thinking harsh punishment is the only answer. If we can step away for a bit, take a deep breath, and respond with curiosity instead of anger, it can create space for our girls to explain or correct themselves. If we quickly resort to threats or punishments, they're likely to become defensive and stick to their story, perpetuating the situation and making it even harder to climb out of the hole.

Every semester, I ask my college students a few questions, starting with, "How many of you are afraid of your parents?" Typically, about half of the class raises their hand. Then I follow up with, "Did that fear prevent you from doing things wrong, or did it simply teach you to conceal your actions better?" Their response is always knowing laughter, indicating that they've indeed become adept at hiding things. Some even admit to feeling driven to rebel against their parents because of the fear they experience or because they felt misunderstood or unseen.

The second question I ask is what they wish for the most when it comes to their parents, and for ten years it's basically been the same: *I wish I could talk to them without feeling afraid. I wish they would get to know me.*

REPAIR

Disagreements, fights, or what clinicians often call "ruptures" typically involve three key elements: *what happened, how we responded,* and *how we see ourselves after it's over.* The event itself, which is what happened, ranges from minor misunderstandings to bigger issues, like our daughter skipping school or getting a speeding ticket.

After the event, our reaction, or how we responded, is influenced by our emotions, past experiences, and coping mechanisms. We may be angry, say unkind or inappropriate things, or completely withdraw and use the silent treatment. It all depends on our history, current stress level, and underlying beliefs about the situation's severity.

Then it's how we feel about ourselves after it's over. An event may lead us to question ourselves, our child, or societal norms, all leading to feelings of incompetence, unworthiness, or loss of control. This can leave us feeling insecure, inadequate, or ashamed as parents. The issue ends up being about more than just the disagreement—it's also about how we see ourselves and our identity.

One of the hardest, yet most necessary, aspects of being a parent is the ability to apologize to our daughters if we hurt or offend them, or if things go off the rails. As the parent and the adult in the relationship, it's our responsibility to model how to own mistakes and take accountability for our actions. Taking a break or taking time to collect ourselves can help us regain our balance, and then it's important to address the harm we've caused, whether it was intentional or accidental.

Instead of debating whether our daughters are justified in feeling upset or offended by something we did, we can believe them when they express their hurt. Even if our intentions were good and not meant to cause harm, if they received them negatively, we need to trust what they are telling us. Just because something wouldn't have bothered us doesn't mean it won't offend or hurt them.

We're all different, and we experience social interactions and the world differently, so our behaviors and experiences won't always align. The key is to learn as much as we can about the people we love when they share what hurts or helps them.

If we neglect to circle back and repair when our daughters are upset or offended, it creates a communication gap. Left unaddressed, they might start blaming themselves for whatever happened. They might not voice this feeling immediately, but eventually, they'll internalize responsibility for unresolved conflicts, much like the way young children blame themselves for their parents' divorce or financial struggles. Repairing these rifts in the relationship allows our girls to reshape their memory of the disagreement. Instead of dwelling on the pain and doubt, they'll remember feeling heard and understood once it was resolved.

Responsibility

Even if something happened a while back and it's still bothering our daughter, we can revisit the issue and take responsibility for our actions. This gives them a chance to rewrite the narrative of what occurred. Instead of holding onto the pain and letting it impact every conversation, they can let go of the burden.

When my oldest daughter Jacey was two, my husband dressed up as Cookie Monster for her birthday. She was terrified when he walked down the stairs, and she wanted him to leave immediately. While the other kids enjoyed his presence as he messily ate cookies, Jacey would not go near him for the entire party.

Before bed that night, she kept asking, "Why you be Cookie Monster?" and she asked again the next morning. We kept telling her how much she loved Cookie Monster and how the other kids were so entertained by him. She wasn't buying it, and for the next year—I'm not exaggerating—she would ask at least once a week, "Why you be Cookie Monster?" One morning, I was so tired, and I knew I needed to say something new, so I said, "We made a big mistake. We shouldn't have had Cookie Monster at your party. You were scared, and we should have listened to you immediately. I am so sorry we did that on your birthday." She thought for a bit, nodded, and never brought it up again.

My husband and I learned a lot from this experience. This is a story about a little girl who was willing to keep articulating her curiosity and pain, but older girls experience the same type of confusion and hurt when a parent emotionally injures them or fails to understand them. Unlike toddlers, they may choose to stop bringing up their feelings because they've learned it leads to nothing, and the continued disappointment is too much for them to handle.

No matter our age or gender, when someone hurts us, we carry that pain, questioning why our feelings or fears weren't considered. Some people in this world never apologize or acknowledge their wrongdoing, and there are those who will intentionally hurt our girls and even blame them. As parents and trusted adults, we can take responsibility for our actions and be mindful of our daughters' feelings, buffering them from some of the shame and blame situations they will inevitably encounter in the world.

While we can't control everything that will happen to them, we can establish a norm within our home for taking accountability. This strengthens their self-confidence and teaches them about the importance of responsibility, helping them develop healthy skills to navigate adult relationships with empathy and trust.

Repair within the home is important for healthy family relationships, and it serves as a counterbalance to instances when our daughters' experiences are dismissed in society. I hear so many stories from girls about being teased or getting unwanted attention from a guy at school, only for adults to dismiss the behavior by attributing it to the boy "liking her" or simply as typical behavior for boys, excusing the actions as normal.

Some girls are advised to simply ignore mistreatment, which implies that it's somehow acceptable. Some adults may even suggest that she provoked it, asking if she'd been flirting or somehow brought it upon herself. Others might downplay the seriousness of the situation, telling her to toughen up and disregarding her fear and discomfort. These are just a few examples of why accountability within the home, specifically our ability to acknowledge and repair our mistakes, models a better foundational understanding of healthy communication for our daughters. It also shows them how to take responsibility for themselves and prepares them for healthy adult relationships.

Good apologies are necessary when we want to repair, and they also serve as valuable lessons for our girls, teaching them the importance of acknowledging when they've hurt someone or crossed a boundary. When apologizing, we should avoid using "but" statements—*I'm sorry I hurt you, but you hurt me first*—because it diminishes the sincerity of our apology and makes it sound like we are making insincere excuses. The goal is to take full accountability for our actions, demonstrating that we understand that we've hurt them. Rather than shifting blame, we focus on acknowledging what we did and expressing a genuine desire to learn and improve.

Somatics and Embodiment

Somatic therapy differs from cognitive-behavioral therapy (CBT) and other talk therapies by focusing on the body, emphasizing how awareness and movement can lead to emotional release and shift thinking. Consulting with a qualified somatic therapist is helpful for better understanding clinical implications and outcomes. Still, I'm including a discussion of somatic understanding and embodiment in this section because it's something our girls seem to understand but need more support in practicing.

Somatics is the understanding of how emotions, stress, and trauma impact our bodies, often resulting in physical discomfort and negative effects on our mental well-being. Techniques involving movement and mindfulness can help release stuck emotions, helping to alleviate both physical and mental stress.

Embodiment means being tuned into your body, feeling its sensations, emotions, and movements in real time. It's about understanding how physical experiences relate to thoughts and feelings, becoming more present in the body, and living life informed by what it feels.

Young women are more aware of somatics and how movement and body awareness can benefit them, thanks in part to platforms like TikTok and YouTube. For years, my college students have been especially interested in Bessel Van der Kolk's teachings from *The Body Keeps the Score* and Gabor Maté's insights into how trauma resides in the body. Social media platforms are not known for sharing the most accurate research when it comes to clinical issues, but they do contribute to a growing awareness of how emotions can manifest physically.

Girls' physical complaints are sometimes dismissed as exaggeration or something they should ignore, especially by their parents, but their aches and pains are real and often connected to their thoughts and experiences. Stomachaches before a test or a headache after an argument are examples of how our emotional experiences can manifest physically in our bodies, and questioning these feelings or telling our girls to stop feeling this way isn't helpful.

Instead of ignoring our girls' physical complaints, we can encourage them to pay attention to their bodies. This helps them identify where they feel pain and understand how and whether it's linked to their emotions. Recognizing these distress signals not only helps our daughters understand the mind/body connection, but also reminds them that they can use self-soothing techniques such as breathing, movement, or taking a break outside, away from their phones, to feel better.

Over time, societal pressures, trauma, and cultural expectations disconnect girls from their bodies, prioritizing thinking over tuning into their physicality. As a result, they struggle to trust their instincts or recognize the signals their body sends. This leads them to over-rely on advice from others or conform to perceived norms instead of knowing, or trusting, what they need.

Body sensitivity is needed for our well-being because it connects us to our intuition and decision-making abilities. We know our sensitivities are diminishing when we prioritize others' opinions or constantly ask everyone else for advice. I see this in the girls and women I work with who don't know what their favorite music is, have daily struggles over what to wear, or have no clear idea of how to spend their free time. Instead, they stay busy and productive, prioritizing what society tells them makes them worthy.

There was a year when one of my daughters struggled with decision-making at school. Instead of listening to what she really wanted and what her body was telling her, she was committed to a rational, data-driven approach, focusing on what she thought she should be doing and what others were telling her to do. Throughout that year, she was sick at least once a month. Eventually, she had to make significant changes, aligning herself with what truly mattered to her, and once she did, her health began to stabilize.

Understanding our body's signals isn't always straightforward; sometimes, there are mixed messages or complete lack of clarity about what we are feeling. Our culture favors quick fixes, but our ability to sit with feelings—even when it's uncomfortable—and take the time to consider and process them is how we figure out what is right for us.

Stretching, yoga, deep breathing, and meditation are all effective ways to release tension and stay in tune with our bodies. These practices don't require a lot of time; a few stretches in the morning, a deep breath before a meal, or a few minutes of meditation with eyes closed before starting the day can reconnect us with ourselves. We often neglect these practices because we think we don't have enough time or worry about doing them wrong. But it literally takes a few minutes a day to reconnect with ourselves, and the more we do it, the more natural it becomes.

As a yoga teacher, I focus a lot on posture, and notice how many young girls are constantly hunched over, whether to hide their developing bodies, engage with their phones, or cope with overwhelming emotions. I always gently remind them to breathe deeply, lift their shoulders up and back, and lift their chin to give them a new perspective and a more empowered way of walking through the world.

Creating a family culture around these practices helps our girls integrate them meaningfully into their lives. They notice when we suggest yoga or meditation classes for them, yet fail to participate ourselves. While we encourage or insist on our girls' growth, we remain stuck in our preferred routines, neglecting to model new behaviors. To teach them emotional awareness and body connection, we can lead by example and demonstrate a willingness to explore.

ADAPT

Girls tell me about the various environments and expectations they navigate, from school and sports to interactions with friends and family, often dealing with scenarios like divorce or family conflicts. Every day, they encounter numerous situations that demand adaptation, which leaves them feeling drained and exhausted. This is just one of the many reasons they may retreat to their rooms when they come home.

As our girls navigate through the demands of school, extracurricular activities, and work, they're expected to easily adapt. Each academic year is like starting over for them, and while some aspects—like friendships, neighborhoods, and family—may remain consistent, expectations change rapidly between school years. If your daughter is forced to find a new friend group, which can be so difficult, or deal with changing schools or multiple living arrangements, the challenges intensify. On top of this, they are all undergoing body and mind changes as they confront expectations regarding behavior, workload, and societal norms.

My Latina and Black clients and students also share their experiences with code-switching, where they feel compelled to adjust their behavior depending on the context. They may modify their speech or conversation topics to align with various settings, which may entail switching between languages like Spanish and English, or adapting their dialect to match their audience. They sense the necessity to tailor their communication styles, transitioning from a relaxed and informal demeanor with friends and family to adopting a more formal tone in academic or professional environments. They lead their lives with a special kind of vigilance, constantly assessing their surroundings and adjusting accordingly in each situation.

As adults, we forget the pressures of being young, assuming that our lives are inherently more stressful or demanding. We have limited memories of how challenging it is to manage a school day—the constant interacting with others, prolonged periods of sitting, adherence to strict rules, social expectations, and academic pressures.

We perceive their days as manageable because we've already been through youth, which leads us to underestimate its difficulty and significance. But for our daughters, this is their entire experience of life. They feel tremendous pressure to excel in every aspect, convinced that their grades, looks, and likability determine their worth as human beings. Lacking enough life experience to think otherwise, they constantly compare themselves to others, adapting as needed to gain acceptance or appreciation.

Expectations

We need to recognize the importance of adapting alongside our daughters, reminding ourselves to remain flexible and responsive as their needs and circumstances evolve. They may have many years invested in a particular sport, dance, or club, only to reach a point where they feel it's no longer fulfilling, or they need a break or something new. If we insist that they're quitting, or resort to guilt or shame tactics to keep them in their current activity, we're failing to listen and adapt.

While our intention may be to act in the best interests of our daughters and support their success, we can also notice when our actions are driven solely by our own needs. We need to acknowledge the possibility that it's us who will miss the socialization or sense of importance associated with our daughter's activity, and we are hesitant to let go of this role. It's possible that we've constructed a vision of her future centered around involvement in a particular sport or activity, and we struggle when she deviates from the path we envisioned.

Girls talk to me about feeling pressure to pursue certain activities because of family expectations. They might feel like they must dance because their mom did, play soccer because their brother does, or join student council because their dad insists it's essential for leadership. But what's missing from the mix is their own voice. There's not enough focus on what they want to do, and too much on what we think they should do. This can drown out their inner authority or make them question their own desires, preventing them from learning their own important life lessons.

As a college professor of social work, I encounter students who are from different departments, but enroll in my class as an elective. At some point in the semester, some share their secret desire to pursue a career in social work, psychology, social justice, or another helping profession, but they tell me that their parents are opposed to this choice, advising them to pursue fields like business or finance for financial stability and a specific career trajectory.

What is overlooked is the fundamental aspect of career and life satisfaction: the genuine desire to pursue something that feels right and makes us excited to attend class, seek internships, or pursue a career aligned with our true selves. When we urge our children to follow in our career footsteps or deny them the opportunity to explore their own interests, we not only limit their career options but also disconnect them from themselves.

The reality is that there are no guarantees in either path. The modern work environment differs significantly from when we were in school. Maintaining employment today is less about grades and degrees and more about emotional intelligence to navigate working with people, as well as creativity and adaptability to keep evolving as the environment changes. Working in this type of landscape is much easier—and more fulfilling—if we genuinely enjoy what we do. When we're stuck in jobs solely for financial gain, rather than pursuing fulfilling careers, we sacrifice the opportunity to live a life that feels like us.

The women I work with who are in midlife often express regret for not listening to themselves and pursuing what they love. Choosing to not pursue piano, design, writing—I've heard every story. They remain frustrated that they sacrificed their passions for what was considered expected or safe. I encourage them to return to the things they love, to worry less about seeking permission or competing with others, and to focus more on simply enjoying what brings them joy. This is not only beneficial for them, it also serves as great behavior-modeling for their daughters.

The things our girls love may evolve into their careers, or just remain lifelong hobbies. It's less about figuring out how everything will work ahead of time, and more about recognizing their passions as integral parts of their identity—parts they are eager to pursue and share with us. As they show interest in new things, it's our curiosity that demonstrates our care, and our ability to adapt to their evolving helps them develop confidence in themselves.

Our girls aren't expected to maintain the same interests throughout life. They may adore something when they're young but eventually outgrow it. Our willingness to support their evolving interests helps them feel more comfortable and accepting of their ever-changing selves.

Even if they develop interests in things we don't fully understand or endorse—like spending money at Sephora, listening to the newest recording artist that we just don't get, creating videos for social media, or researching tattoos—our ability to engage with their interests by asking questions, and even asking them to include us somehow, keeps us close.

When we approach them with interest instead of criticism or demands, they are more likely to seek our opinion and understand our boundaries. Simply telling them they're wrong or criticizing their choices pushes them away, leaving them to seek validation and acknowledgment elsewhere.

See

In Zen Buddhism, it's taught that if we simply name something, like a tree, we miss out on truly experiencing the tree. But if we observe a tree without the word *tree*, we find it fascinating and unique. Similarly, when we see our daughters beyond just their grades or extracurricular activities, we open ourselves up to experiencing them in a new light—as intriguing, interesting people. This helps us see them as they are, instead of as who we expect them to be.

Many of the girls I work with struggle with depression and anxiety, often due to the pressure they feel and their inability to pursue their passions or engage in activities that truly matter to them. They feel compelled to invest time and energy in things that don't align with their interests, which leaves them feeling drained.

What they are doing is prioritizing others' needs over their own, and it's causing their inspiration to fade and their sense of self to diminish. It leaves them lost in the pursuit of *perfection, pleasing, and proving*—a mindset that many find difficult to untangle until midlife, if they are lucky.

Girls want to share their poetry and hope adults will listen without rejecting their dreams as irresponsible just because they might not be profitable. They want to explore politics and law without hearing discouraging remarks about the challenges of balancing motherhood with a high-profile career. As parents, we are often too focused on practicalities, instead of allowing our girls to discover themselves through trying, failing, and exploring.

As our daughters grow up and begin dressing more maturely, going out alone, or taking on driving responsibilities, it's important for us to continuously adjust our expectations and maintain open, approachable conversations with them. By recognizing and treating them according to their actual age rather than getting stuck in time, we demonstrate that we are paying attention and that we are excited about their growth. It's important that they not feel guilty about growing up; it's challenging enough for them without feeling like they're letting down their parents.

The girls I work with in therapy sessions want to share what they feel and experience with their parents, but they sense that their parents don't really want to see them; they would rather see what they expect them to be. There is no room for the girls' hopes, dreams, fears, and questions because their parents' expectations have already filled up these spaces.

If the girl wants to maintain a relationship with her parents, she feels she must conform to these expectations, or at least pretend to do so in their presence. This is when she starts to distance herself, adjusting her behavior depending on the people she's with, and prioritizing others over herself.

LGBTQ+

The current political climate can further complicate discussions and create fear around self-exploration, specifically when it comes to sexuality and gender. I have worked with young people exploring their sexuality and gender identity for over twenty years. Despite societal conversation portraying identity exploration as new or trendy, I can assure you that queer curiosity and identity are not novel concepts. There's just more space and acceptance to discuss things openly.

The suicide rate among LGBTQ+ youth is higher because there is a fear of rejection or being disowned by their families, and unfortunately, some experience this reality. My oldest daughter identifies as gay and she has shared with me the experience of internalized homophobia, even being in our family, which is open and accepting. She swims in a culture that questions and judges, which made her question and judge herself. And even with our support, she still had to do a lot of internal work to accept herself fully.

Maybe your daughter has already discussed her sexuality or gender with you, but even if she hasn't, know that learning and exploration take up a lot of space in her mind and heart. This is another opportunity for us to tap into a young person's perspective, to remember how much we thought about attraction and sex at their age, especially before we'd had any experiences.

Your daughter may identify as straight and cisgender (gender identity matches the sex they were assigned at birth), or there may be a curiosity about or identification with queerness. Regardless, the fear of not being accepted or loved is profound and vulnerable, so it's critical to convey to our daughters that we are there for them as their self-awareness unfolds.

We need to assure them, both through words and actions, that we are open to adapting and learning, and that we are steadfast in our support. We shouldn't assume that we already know how they identify or ask them solely about boys or boyfriends. Using language about partnership or attraction offers a broader perspective, indicating that we simply want them to find relationships that are meaningful to them.

There was a time when I attended church with my daughters, and after every service that included a sermon, I'd make sure to retell the intended message at home, ensuring its inclusivity and removing anything hinting at exclusivity. I spent so many services strategizing how to convey every sermon to my girls in a way that emphasized love and support for all people. Then, one week, a guest speaker referred to Mary Magdalene as the "whore at the well," and I knew I had hit my limit. I found myself questioning why I was subjecting myself and my daughters to sermons that I then had to reinterpret at home with empathy and inclusivity.

That's when we stopped attending and explored new avenues for spiritual practice. I know that not all churches are the same; there are plenty that embrace and preach a more inclusive approach. But in our situation at the time, it was clear that the essence of the message was being distorted by the messenger. I worried that, over time, my girls would hear or sense the underlying negative interpretations of womanhood or sexuality, and I feared they would internalize them, making it hard to undo. I can't protect them from all the messaging in the world, but I can be thoughtful about what I am bringing into their lives and what I am validating as okay.

Even if our girls gravitate toward more traditional identities and attractions, they will inevitably have friends who identify differently. Depending on where you live or the school your daughter attends, she may have a diverse group of friends and acquaintances. It's important to create an emotionally safe environment within the home and to get to know the people who are significant in their lives. By doing so, we can become an additional source of comfort for those closest to our girls, offering a space where everyone feels recognized, welcomed, and safe to be themselves.

Denying or avoiding our girls' exploration doesn't prevent them from discovering who they truly are. They are inherently driven to understand themselves, despite any fears or uncertainties they may feel at home that might lead them to pretend or withhold information. Eventually, they will reach a point where they realize they must prioritize themselves, whether it's in high school, in college, or later in life—and we either adapt and support them or miss the chance to truly know them.

A GUIDE FOR REAL CONVERSATIONS

LEAD

One of the girls I work with told me that, for a long time, she would come home from school and tell her parents she was feeling depressed. She said that sometimes her parents would give her a quick hug, or point out why things are actually good, and then do their best to change the subject. This girl decided to experiment with different words and say she was feeling anxious, overwhelmed, or stressed, to see if it would elicit a different response, but the more she tried to articulate her feelings, the more her parents seemed to avoid the conversation.

When I finally spoke to her parents, they acknowledged that they had heard what she was saying, but assumed it was typical teenage behavior or just attention-seeking. Parents often seem to think that attention-seeking is something they can disregard, but teenagers seek attention for valid reasons, and they often need help.

When it comes to depression, people don't pretend to be depressed; they're much more likely to pretend that they are okay, so hearing that someone feels depressed means they need support. As I talked to these parents more about this, they opened up about their own fears, admitting that diving deeper into what their daughter was saying felt overwhelming and intimidating, and they were hesitant to explore where it might lead.

Sometimes, when we anticipate a difficult conversation or issue on the horizon, we focus more on managing the situation than on directly addressing it. We do whatever it takes to convince ourselves that a conversation isn't necessary, seeking confirmation from wherever we can find it and gathering knowledge that aligns with our beliefs. Instead of simply asking the difficult questions or confronting things head-on, all our energy gets directed toward convincing ourselves that this conversation isn't needed.

On the other side of this issue, some parents ask far too many questions, hovering around their child's door, desperate to know every detail of their emotional state. This behavior is less about meaningful conversation and more about the parent trying to calm their own insecurity or anxiety. It's a desire to anticipate any problem to avoid any uncomfortable surprises.

We've all likely fallen into both patterns—avoiding conversations at times, and at other times coming on too strong. These are again examples of how things get messy, and our ability to recognize when we're doing either extreme creates an opening to try a different approach. Initiating discussions about topics that might challenge our perceptions of our children or the world can feel daunting, as if everything is spinning out of control. It's understandable to want to sidestep this discomfort, but in doing so, we invest the same amount of time and energy in avoiding the issue as we would in working toward addressing it.

When we observe shifts in our girls' behavior, or when they openly share painful feelings or challenges with us, it's not necessarily a reason to panic. It's just a signal that we need to pay closer attention and become more aware of what's happening. With time, we start recognizing patterns in their behavior—for example, they might feel more depressed at the beginning of a school year or more anxious at the start of a sports season.

When we begin to observe and understand the ebb and flow of their experiences, we can normalize these patterns in our minds. But when we notice something that raises concern or seems different, it's our responsibility to take the lead and ask questions. We shouldn't assume that our daughters know how to effectively communicate their needs to us.

I can't count the number of times a parent has said to me, "My daughter knows she can come to me if she's struggling," but when I work with the daughter, she doesn't know that. She doesn't feel safe, or she is concerned that whatever she shares will alter the relationship. Sometimes she wants to protect herself from hurt, and other times she's trying to shield her parent, and either way, she feels too scared to share. This reluctance to share usually leads our girls to depend on their peers for information, and while their peers can be loving and supportive, they still lack the maturity or resources to offer helpful advice.

Alternative Solutions

When my oldest daughter was young, she told me that telling me things was difficult because she didn't want to see my eyes change. I had no idea what this meant, but instead of arguing with her about what she was noticing, we came up with a plan to have her write things to me in a notebook. Whenever she wanted to tell me something big, she wrote it down and then threw it on my bed. I would write back and put it back on her bed, and from that point on, we were usually safe to engage in a face-to-face discussion. Now that the difficult things were said, my eyes were less likely to show any big shifts in emotion.

This method worked all the way through high school and beyond. Over the years, through writing, she told us she identified as gay, shared the mental health challenges of some of her friends who were really struggling, and expressed the things that made her feel scared or ashamed. To this day, she still writes letters to me on Mother's Day, writes her dad a letter on his birthday, and shares letters with her sisters and friends on big occasions. She found a way to share her feelings without the overwhelm of the other person's experience and emotion, and she still utilizes it today to stay connected.

Leading a conversation means being open to solutions like this that may be different than what we are used to. A good leader doesn't insist on a single approach; they focus on understanding people's personalities and skill sets, allowing them to shine or contribute in their own unique way. The way our daughters communicate as children will likely evolve as they grow into teenagers or young adults. Our ability to adapt and find new methods of communication, rather than becoming fixated on a specific approach, allows us to stay connected as they navigate more vulnerable situations and develop their own communication style.

Some parents tend to carry a vision in their mind of how things should play out, and anything less than that feels like not enough. Rather than simply appreciating a heartfelt text from their daughter that reads, "I love you!" they might wonder why she doesn't express it more in person. They might enjoy a meaningful conversation with their daughter during the car ride home from a soccer tournament, only to feel frustrated that such discussions don't occur nightly around the dinner table. At times, we lose sight of what truly matters, opting instead to exert control over situations or fixate on ensuring they unfold exactly as we envision every time.

Leadership in conversations also involves granting permission for our daughters to communicate with and depend on people other than us. We can play a key role in building a supportive community for them, ensuring they know who they can rely on. When each of my daughters turned thirteen, I organized a party to celebrate their growth and transition into their teenage years. The guest list included the women in my life who were most important to me and whom I trusted to support my daughters.

At the party, each of the guests wrote letters and read them aloud, and they shared symbolic gifts to remind my daughters to stay true to themselves. The idea was to create a community where my girls felt comfortable reaching out to any of these women, and where they felt they belonged to a community that cared about them.

Over the years, my daughters have relied on these women, expanding their circle to include other trusted adults. My youngest sought support from her school counselor during a tough time, my middle daughter received her first job offer from a close family friend, and my oldest developed an ongoing, valued relationship with one of my favorite work friends, who she even asked to write her college recommendation letter.

Not only is this beneficial for them, but as a mom, I feel less alone. While I still see myself as the frontline of defense, inevitably carrying the greatest concern and responsibility for my daughters' well-being, whenever they face significant challenges, I also encourage the caring women in their lives to reach out to them and encourage my daughters to reach out to these women. This not only makes my daughters and me feel supported, it also exposes them to a diverse range of female role models and various life paths for their own future.

Emotional Release

There have been times when my daughters wanted to discuss something important late at night, and while I try my best to listen so they can express what they need in that moment, I also let them know that I might not be at my best. Like most parents, at night, I'm so tired that I don't feel like I can be an effective listener. This is when I commit to creating a plan to continue this discussion, emphasizing how important it is to me. Sometimes I suggest breakfast together the next morning or spending time together after school.

It's quite common for our daughters to finally open up to us at night, sharing their emotions and struggles at school, frustrations with teachers, or feelings of loneliness. Nighttime tends to be a vulnerable time for all of us, when our defenses are lowered and we can emotionally unload. When your daughters share their thoughts and feelings with you at night, their goal is not to be difficult or hard on you. They're simply experiencing a moment when their guard is down, allowing them to share everything that's been on their mind throughout the day, including their fears and insecurities. Their feelings are genuine, but it's more of an unfiltered emotional release than an accurate reflection of their daily reality.

A parent recently shared with me an experience where her daughter confided in her about various school concerns late one night, prompting this mom to call the school the next morning to address these issues. But the school had no knowledge of what she was talking about, saying her daughter actually has a lot of friends and acclimates quite well.

When the mom told her daughter she'd made this call, her daughter was so embarrassed, because she didn't actually need that kind of assistance— she simply needed to unload her feelings. There's a distinction between being there for our girls as they express their emotions, and taking action. While there are times when action is necessary, often our girls just need a safe space to vent, especially late at night when they feel most open.

If this is a common occurrence with your daughter, consider giving it a name, like "end of the day unloading" or "nighttime emotional release." Treat it seriously and respectfully, acknowledging its importance. This process allows our daughters to clear some emotional space within themselves so they can face the next day with clarity. We're there to listen, but we don't have to carry the weight of their feelings.

Sometimes, when my daughters or even a client shares a lot of information, I'll open a window to create a type of emotional ventilation. It can be seen as a metaphorical concept, referring to the process of releasing emotions or thoughts to reduce psychological tension and stress. We can also use candles, incense, or other symbolic gestures to signify that something significant is being shared and that we are preparing the space for it.

We need to remember that knowing our girls are in pain, or hearing them talk about what hurts, also feels painful for us. Naturally, feeling our own pain demonstrates our care for our girls, but when we experience heightened pain that seems disproportionate, it's often a sign of our own unresolved past pain being projected onto our daughters' current situation.

For example, if our daughter shares that she doesn't have any friends to sit with at lunch, we may have an overblown reaction because it brings up times when we didn't have any friends to sit with at lunch. We are no longer present; we are feeling our history. My sister-in-law is in recovery, and one of her favorite AA wisdoms that applies here is *if you're hysterical, it's historical.*

Overblown reactions tend to go one of two ways: either we get too intense and worried, which tells our daughter she should indeed worry about this problem and that we are just as upset about it as she is, making us unable to really offer any help; or we have a denial response where we try to downplay or avoid it because we don't want to feel the pain, maybe even telling our daughter that she is overreacting or weak for even being bothered.

It's important to carve out space between our history and what is happening with our girls in present time, making sure we recognize what is theirs and what is ours. We don't need to take on what they feel; we just need to recognize their perspective and be with them as they feel it. We need to believe them when they tell us they are in pain and, at the same time, trust that they have what it takes to move through the pain. Pain, like all things, is a cycle, and our girls can move through it if they have space to share without fearing shame or judgment.

Big feelings, or unspoken pain, are like an internal dirty window, clouding the way we see the world. Once something is shared with someone we trust, it's a natural window cleaning, allowing some light to shine through. When our girls share their most significant fears and worries with us, and then they end with a good cry or laugh, they tend to conclude the conversation with a more enlightened understanding, like, "Well, this is definitely hard, but I'm actually okay." Not because what they shared wasn't real, but because releasing heavy feelings helped them balance their emotional and rational mind, allowing them to feel more grounded and safer.

As we guide our daughters through these moments, we play an important role in keeping communication open. We can consider what it's like to be in their shoes, instead of deciding that what they are experiencing is overblown. We can validate their experiences, giving them the freedom to explore every emotion, rather than rejecting them. Therapists call this "creating space"—stepping back to let many viewpoints emerge and allow the full picture to unfold. By doing this, we help our daughters clear their own path, so they gain a better understanding of themselves moving forward.

Initiate

When I talk about being us being the leaders, I mean specifically that we're willing to initiate conversations and check in about the big conversations we've already had. When we take the lead on important conversations—especially the ones we might want to avoid but realize are vital—we're giving our girls more than just our attention; we're modeling valuable skills for handling the challenges of interacting with other people. They learn how to approach difficult conversations courageously and how to handle them with compassion and humility.

A GUIDE FOR REAL CONVERSATIONS

By setting this example, we're empowering our girls to become not just effective communicators, but kind and empathetic people.

Starting difficult conversations can feel intimidating, but we can approach them with a sense of openness and curiosity rather than strict expectations. Asking open-ended questions and giving our girls space when they share their discomfort is helpful. Giving space doesn't mean fully disengaging; it means maintaining our composure and considering another way. The calmer we are, the safer our daughters will feel to keep talking. If they pause or seem unsure, we can gently prompt them with questions like:

- "Tell me more about..."
- "How did you handle that...?"
- "Help me understand the last thing you said..."
- "I'm curious about how you are feeling now..."

We can respond to statements with:

- "That makes sense."
- "I'm glad you can talk about this."
- "Good for you."
- "I'm sorry that happened."
- "If you need me, let me know."

Low-key questions and supportive responses, which are not demanding but just gentle and curious, can help continue a difficult conversation when we notice our girls are backing off or starting to feel uncomfortable. To decrease their discomfort, we need to improve our ability to manage our own discomfort, and do our best to stay engaged even when the conversation becomes unexpected. Again, messiness and mistakes are normal, and sometimes being the leader of a conversation means pausing and restarting later, maybe five minutes later, or even waiting until the next day.

BE LIGHT

Instead of discussing challenges and having real conversations about how the world can be unsafe, unkind, or unfair, parents sometimes demonstrate or act out these negative possibilities in the home to teach their girls lessons. One mother I worked with made her daughter walk home, alone, late at night, because the car had run out of gas, and it was the daughter's job to fill up the tank. Mom insisted that this real-world approach would make an impact, which it did, but it also made her daughter feel unsafe and untrusting of her mom. If we become the harm that we're trying to shield our girls from, we may be inadvertently teaching them that they can't count on others for help.

In just one school day, our girls encounter a multitude of people, disappointments, fears, and anxieties, offering them a daily crash course in life's trials. Rather than adding to this already overwhelming mix, we can be the people who help them navigate what's difficult, openly discussing challenges and figuring out ways to overcome them. This way, we alleviate their burdens, rather than adding to them.

There was a recent viral video featuring Michelle Obama where she said she doesn't want to become friends with her daughters because then she would have to worry about being liked. She explained that her daughters need to hear no in the home so they can handle no in the world, and that disappointment is expected and part of the parenting experience. These are valid points—establishing rules, boundaries, and structures is essential for creating a safe foundation for our girls, and of course we will sometimes need to say no when they are not emotionally or developmentally ready for an experience.

We can balance this by understanding that we can also be friendly with our girls. We can establish rules without being jerks, have expectations without being overbearing, and create structure without being scary. Again, the way we build a relationship with them serves as a template for their future relationships and how they perceive the world. Do they fear authority or respect it? Do they resort to fighting and insults to communicate, or do they engage in discussions, listen, and empathize?

From my personal and professional experience, I've learned that maintaining a sense of friendliness with our girls makes it much easier to share our opinions and set limits. If a parent-daughter relationship is enjoyable and valued, there's less desire to harm it. Our girls will be more likely to experience guilt, not want to disappoint, and tell the truth rather than lie. But if they constantly feel angry at us, or don't feel that we respect or understand them, it's easier for them to push us away, do things behind our backs, and care less about what we think.

Connecting with our girls in a way that prioritizes the relationship over their performance is a preventative measure. Even when they're testing boundaries, they'll be more open to hearing our reasons for saying no and more likely to trust that we're looking out for their safety.

One of my favorite books about writing is *Writing Down the Bones* by Natalie Goldberg. In one chapter, she advises being specific and precise with writing, and in the next chapter she suggests letting go of control. Another chapter suggests setting up a studio and making it a favorite writing space, and the next chapter encourages writing in new places.

This writing paradox is like parenting—it's a blend of structure, seriousness, flexibility, and silliness. We establish boundaries and expectations, yet within the same day, a conversation with our girls might prompt us to reconsider a rule and devise a completely new strategy. We could have a heartfelt discussion one moment, then find ourselves singing along to songs in the car together just thirty minutes later. It's a constant ebb and flow, characterized by gray areas and no one-size-fits-all solutions. This uncertainty leads us to frequently second-guess ourselves, which is also to be expected.

It's why teaching, podcasting, or writing about parenting can be so tough—because it's nuanced, always changing, and it calls for different parts of ourselves at different times. There's no standardized approach; it's all about adapting to the individual and being ready to pivot in the moment, rather than rigidly sticking to a predetermined plan. Parenting is about being human.

Pebbling

In the morning, I might give my daughter a hug and tell her about my dream. Or maybe I'll talk to her about the latest Taylor Swift song or reminisce about an inside joke from *Parks & Rec* or the Twilight movies. She may share her thoughts about a Taylor Jenkins-Reid book she's reading for the third time, and we like to discuss how great the music is in *Daisy Jones and the Six*.

I text my daughters in college lots of funny reels, articles, capybara pictures, or updates on our pet rabbit. On our family group text, we share updates about Mike Flanagan's latest series, the release dates for the next season of *Yellowjackets* or *Severance*, or an old family picture along with some kind of inside joke. I recently learned that this behavior is called "pebbling," inspired by penguins gifting pebbles to potential partners. Sending memes, links, and videos signals that you are thinking of someone and want to share your joy with them. Every pebble is an attempt to connect.

I saw a lavender chai latte on the menu while eating brunch the other day, so I took a picture of it and texted it to my daughter, who loves lavender chai, and she responded, "Must get!" Before I started writing this chapter, I sent all three girls a screenshot of the lineup for this year's Lollapalooza and asked if they planned to attend and, if so, who they were going to see. Sometimes, when my daughter walks in the door from school, to be funny, Todd and I will stand up and start clapping, and Todd will say, "There she is!"

I work with a mom who puts notes in her daughter's lunches to remind her to have a good day, and I know a dad who writes his daughter a letter every Sunday, encouraging her to expect the best and look for the good. Making a point to engage with our girls in ways that have nothing to do with our needs or expectations, or their schedules and grades—but instead are about enjoying each other and being friendly, fun, and human—are deposits in their emotional bank accounts.

Picture our expectations and conflicts as withdrawals from their emotional back accounts. Each time we engage in enjoyable activities, give sincere compliments, or share laughter together, their emotional bank accounts get replenished. This ensures that there's enough to draw from without depleting their emotional resources.

Pebbling can be in simple moments scattered throughout the day, nothing that requires extra time or planning. It's about setting aside the "parent" role to be more sociable and friendly. Through these casual, enjoyable conversations, our girls internalize that we genuinely like them, enjoy talking with them, and appreciate who they are. We build a relationship based on mutual trust, rather than solely on the parent-child dynamic.

Our girls also need hugs, back rubs, or other physically affectionate ways of connecting—whatever soothes them, calms them, and makes them feel loved. As they grow older, they may not seek this as often, but they still need it. The key lies in our ability to offer these gestures without insistence or making them feel guilty for not reciprocating. Even brief acts, like a quick hug or briefly holding their hand, can help calm their nervous systems and create a stronger sense of connection with us.

I have worked with families who needed to start by first engaging in more fun activities, and then gradually reintroducing hugs. Sometimes, a new kind of trust or connection needs to be developed before the girls are open to physical affection, and it's important to respect where they are and what they say they want. But when the opportunity for hugs arises—not just when they're saying goodbye or going to bed, but also when they're hanging around or walking in the door from school—it's another way to remind them that we love having them around and that we're grateful to love them.

Lovability

Continuously asking our girls about their social lives or school achievements can feel like pressure to them. We usually do this to ease our own anxieties by having them recount everything they're doing, leaving us feeling relieved, or allowing us to identify problems we can then focus on. In my experience, our girls usually have a plan and feel in control, knowing they can turn to us for help when necessary, but our constant pressure can disrupt these instincts, potentially leading them to avoid us instead.

Our girls' approach to tasks will often differ from ours, which is to be expected, given our decades of additional experience as adults. Expecting them to be like us or to do things the way we do doesn't make sense. Developing organizational skills takes time and involves learning from experiences, including failure. If we understand this, our daughters are more likely to appreciate it when we offer our support and encouragement. Conversely, if we're constantly annoyed or exasperated by their inability to meet our expectations or do things our way, they're more likely to reject or distance themselves from our help.

If our daughters feel that the level of attention and love we give them is determined by their success and obedience to our demands, it will lead to resentment. In 2014, a study conducted by the Harvard Graduate School of Education found that 80 percent of young people believed their parents cared more about their achievements than about whether they were being kind. Ten years after this study, I continue to hear stories from girls who believe their parents love them more when they get As, only want to engage with them when they have good news, and only notice them when they accomplish something outstanding.

Our ability to connect with our daughters based on who they are, rather than just what they achieve, helps them handle setbacks and feel comfortable seeking support when they need it. If our girls believe that their lovability depends on their achievements and excellence, they will be much less likely to share their challenges because their relationship with us is at stake.

At the heart of our relationship with our daughters is the ability to affirm their value and worth. We can be their support systems, reminding them that they matter, genuinely appreciating them, and celebrating who they are more than what they do. If we don't celebrate who they are at their core, who will?

Projection

When we neglect self-care or fail to pay attention to our own self-awareness, we not only lose track of what might benefit our girls, but we may also end up relying on them to regulate our emotions. Our anxiety or insecurity might prompt us to seek reassurance from them, or when we feel overwhelmed, we may project our feelings of stress onto them, becoming more involved in their lives instead of paying attention to our own.

To alleviate our own discomfort and doubts about ourselves, we might find ourselves pressuring our daughters to excel, to stand out, or always come first, to boost our own self-esteem. Think of those beauty pageants and dance competitions where moms are overly invested, pushing their daughters toward a specific outcome so they can feel better about themselves. It's a subtle form of coercion, guiding our daughters to conform to certain ideals just to validate our own sense of worth.

We might insist that our daughters wear their hair a certain way, or pressure them to wear specific clothes for compliments. We might urge them to join certain clubs or groups we think are important, or coerce them into doing TikToks with us to showcase a close bond or keeping up with trends. In doing so, we sidestep addressing our own issues, and instead place the emotional weight of our lives on our daughters' shoulders. We avoid our own personal growth, expecting our daughters to excel and provide us with a shortcut to feeling good about ourselves.

Being light in our communication style also means being aware of how we show up and allowing our girls to focus on themselves rather than satisfy all our needs. It's about engaging with who they are, rather than telling them who to be. It means focusing on enjoying the small, funny moments with them and appreciating their interests, even if they don't lead to any awards or accolades.

Our ability to create a culture in our homes that includes fun and laughter is what makes a girl want to come home from school and relax, or come home from college and feel comforted, or come home as an adult to enjoy a meal or spend time together. When it comes to being light, much of it is about nurturing a relationship for both the moment and the future, becoming a soft place to land rather than the source of our daughter's greatest stress.

When I teach, I often use the metaphor of a balance beam to explain the parenting journey. At the beginning, we hold our daughter's hand as she walks the beam, offering guidance and protection. But as she grows, we gradually step back, allowing her to develop her own balance and skills. We step back, but we are still readily available to help her get back onto the beam if she falls or gets hurt. Then, we step back again, watching from a distance. Our distance demonstrates that we trust her, and because we're still present and watching, she knows we're available if needed.

If we can be ourselves with our girls, share humor, and have a sense of lightness with them, parenting becomes more enjoyable and increases the likelihood that our girls will want to spend time with us. Instead of switching personalities—acting one way with friends and colleagues while being different, or more serious, with our kids—we can authentically be ourselves in every setting. This allows our girls to know us as people rather than just as parents.

Wonder

To prioritize wonder in our girls' lives, we can illuminate simple joys in our daily routines. This might mean pausing to smell the flowers, feeling the breeze through an open door, observing the busy activity of ants, rabbits, and squirrels, going for walks together, or simply sitting outside to appreciate the trees and listen to the birds' songs. These activities are commonplace when our girls are younger, but as they grow older, we can easily overlook their importance. We need to remember that our girls need reminders to marvel at the world just as much as they did when they were little.

If we consistently appreciate simple things in our surroundings, our daughters will be influenced to do the same. It's normal for teenagers to become less receptive, or even resistant, to noticing nature or other small wonders. Adolescence and young adulthood bring a flood of new thoughts and experiences, understandably causing them to feel more removed from the simple things they loved in their younger years. Even so, we can continue to prioritize this for ourselves, reinforcing to our girls that age doesn't inhibit our ability to notice what's awesome.

Every summer, I make it a tradition to find at least one caterpillar, giving it a name, often after a character from one of our favorite shows. Usually, I'm the one who takes care of it, but we all observe and appreciate its growth as it eventually morphs into a cocoon. When the butterfly emerges, I take it outside on my finger so its wings can dry, then wait until it's ready to fly away. If the girls are home, they help me, and if they aren't, I take pictures and videos and share them in our group chat.

I'm not particularly skilled at gardening, but I make an effort to grow a few things every summer: tomatoes for our dinners and parsley for our rabbit. I have a few house plants that we name (my favorite one is Georgia O'Leaf) and have a lot of signs and sayings around the house that remind us that we can do hard things and to appreciate the good. I enjoy initiating conversations with the girls about the phases of the moon and the movements of the planets, mainly because they often know more than I do, and it's fun when they teach me what they know.

A GUIDE FOR REAL CONVERSATIONS

Last year, we had a squirrel in our front yard with a wounded paw, making him easy to spot every day. We named him Barney, and for over a month, we watched him gracefully navigate the trees and manage to eat with only one paw. He became quite an inspiration to us, reminding us that we are capable of more than we think. We still keep an eye out for him, but now most squirrels we see are lovingly dubbed Barney.

We have three bird feeders on the front tree, and we keep a set of binoculars by the front door so we can observe them up close. We also purchased a bird feeder camera and created a video featuring all the critters that visited. The video included close-up shots of various types of birds and lots of squirrels. What made it even sweeter and funnier to watch was that in the background, you could see all of us coming, going, and sitting on the porch, hanging out with each other, over time.

I once worked with a woman who was navigating through a particularly difficult period with her daughter, and for a while, their days were filled with tension and disagreements. She was able to have a real conversation with her daughter about how uncomfortable their relationship had become and how she really wanted to connect and make things less heavy.

They didn't know what to do to change things, so they just made a pact to share a moment together each night, looking at the stars or admiring the sunset. This ritual was a reminder that there are forces greater than their immediate struggles, putting things in perspective and reminding them to be grateful. Over time, the tension decreased.

For a long time, I kept a coincidence journal, where I wrote down unexpected or meaningful coincidences to track moments where events align in a significant or meaningful ways. I also like to write down my dreams, especially if they are good, and I also write down significant interactions during the day that made me feel good. I have encouraged my girls to do things like this, to have a gratitude journal to remember what's working, or to write down experiences that were helpful, so they don't get lost in the shuffle of a day.

It's important to remember that the top ten headlines of the day do not reflect the complete truth about our world. We can make it a priority to be attentive and notice the positive things that are happening around us because they are always there. Recognizing what works offers a more well-rounded and often appreciative orientation to our lives. It doesn't deny what's difficult or negative; it only highlights what's overlooked or taken for granted.

As Carlos Castañeda, an American anthropologist and writer, famously said, "The aim is to balance the terror of being alive with the wonder of being alive," and this is precisely what makes parenting so amazing and challenging. It's about balancing the realities of everyday life with nurturing wonder and curiosity in our girls, guiding them to live in reality while also exploring deeper, more mysterious aspects of themselves and the world.

CHAPTER 4

Real Things Girls Want You to Know

For over a decade, I've been documenting the things girls most commonly wish their parents knew. During sessions, in workshops, in the college classroom, and even in my own home—girls speak about what bothers them the most or what they wish they could better articulate.

While there are variations in how they express themselves or their specific needs, most of these requests or comments have remained consistent over the years. They represent the things girls wish they could say and wish their parents would understand.

This list is extensive, but not exhaustive, as every girl will have her own unique set of needs based on her own personal experiences. These comments can serve as a starting point. You can ask your daughters if they agree and encourage them to share what they feel is missing.

Reflecting back to the opening of the book—when I mentioned that girls ask me, "Can you please tell my parents this?"—the essence of "this" again includes:

- Will you help them understand who I am so they will *know me*?
- Will you ask them not to shame me or judge me and instead *connect with me*?
- Will you help them become better listeners and *support me*?
- Will you remind them that I am doing my best and to *trust me*?
- Will you tell them to take life less seriously and *laugh with me*?

These are the specifics about what they mean and what they hope we are willing to understand.

KNOW ME

Let Me Tell You about Me, Instead of You Telling Me about Me

Girls get frustrated when they are told who they are and what they should do. When we assume we know more about our girls than they know about themselves, we will immediately run face-first into their understandable defensiveness. As parents, we, of course, believe we know our kids well; we've lived with them, watched them grow, and supported them in innumerable ways. But we must differentiate between what we've observed and what's going on inside of them.

One of the things I learned in my own therapy was that when my daughters were going through difficult experiences, I assumed I understood exactly how they felt and what the outcomes would probably be, based on my own experiences. What my therapist helped me realize is that because my girls' lives have been so different from mine—their upbringing, their generation, even where they lived and with whom—they would not have the exact same perspective as me.

They would see things from their own unique perspective, but I was viewing their experiences only through the lens of my own past. I failed to recognize that they were processing their experiences through their own distinct framework—one shaped by their own strengths, weaknesses, and life circumstances. As a result, they were engaging with everything in an entirely different way than I do. I may be able to relate or have empathy, but I can't assume I literally "know" exactly what they are going through. That's for them to figure out and then tell me, not for me to assume.

Also, our ability to be mindful and refrain from thoughtlessly labeling our daughters as "the smart one," "the athletic one," or even using negative terms like the "flighty" or "dramatic" one, allows them to explore various identities as they grow up. Stepping back and allowing them to pursue multiple paths, instead of insisting on one we've assigned or deemed "right," helps them develop their confidence and self-awareness.

I've had so many girls tell me how they can't stand it when their parents tell them that high school is supposed to be "the best years of their lives" or that college will be "the most fun they ever had." This may not be true for all girls, and these types of declarations end up feeling like pressure, or like they are missing something vital. We need to allow our girls to tell us when they are having the time of their lives, not tell them when they should be. And our romanticized version of our history is probably a bit off the mark; we have forgotten a lot that made it difficult and have tended to cherry-pick what made it exciting.

If we dictate who they are and presume to understand them better than they understand themselves (an idea that might sound noble in books and movies, but is inaccurate in real life), our daughters will eventually need to unlearn and overcome this as they mature. If they learn to rely on us or others more than themselves, they will enter adulthood lacking the ability to make decisions independently, and when we're no longer here, they may feel as if they don't have the wisdom to make their own choices.

Instead of making them put all their faith in us and what we know, we can help them trust in themselves and their own problem-solving skills. We can listen to them attentively and validate their feelings, rather than assuming we always have the right answers.

My Actions Aren't Always about You; I'm Figuring Things Out, Too

Our girls wish we understood that they are creating their own lives, and that their choices or challenges are not always about us. We may tend to cast ourselves as the central figure in every story, and while we play an important role in our daughters' lives, we are rarely the central figure in their decision-making.

We tend to interpret our daughters' actions as a reflection on us—whether they are benefiting or harming us, whether it makes us look good or bad. As parents, our kids are the focal point of our world, but we aren't always the focal point of theirs, nor should we be. They love us, need us, appreciate us, but their actual job is to eventually separate from us and find their own lives. If we have established a positive relationship with them, the bond will evolve, and we will come to appreciate each other as adults, continuing to prioritize family relationships—but this is more likely to happen if, during their formative years, they found us to be people they could talk to and learn from, rather than the people they had to placate or figure out how to work around.

REAL THINGS GIRLS WANT YOU TO KNOW

The hope is that our girls are focused on their own needs and growth, because this is necessary for their progression in the world. Hopefully, they are also learning to be compassionate toward our experiences, and together we've learned how to communicate effectively (which is what this book is for!). This will be dependent on the examples we set in our interactions with them.

The bottom line is that we should focus on nurturing their independence and developing a compassionate and clear way for them to communicate with us. This is achieved through checking in, recognizing and tempering our judgment, and practicing the aspects covered in the previous chapters about real conversations. It's about understanding our role as parents without needing to be at the forefront of every decision they make.

I worked with a fifteen-year-old who lived in constant fear of disappointing her mother. Her mother had struggled during her own teen years and was still learning how to take care of herself in adulthood. She shared a lot of her experiences with her daughter, frequently oversharing and forgetting that she was talking with a young girl rather than a peer. She conveyed to her daughter in various ways that her depression was triggered or exacerbated by any challenges her daughter faced. Consequently, this girl internalized this responsibility, believing that her actions determined her mother's mental well-being.

It's a reminder of how young girls can be easily burdened by the emotional welfare of their parents. I see this primarily with daughters, less so with sons. I especially see this pattern with first-born girls or the daughter who was labeled the "easy one," because she became skilled at putting others before herself. Early on, she internalized the message that her emotions weren't a priority because she needed to show up and help in some way, so she never relied on others to meet her own needs.

The adult women I work with who were first-born or the "easy child" tend to hide behind being overly productive and smiling through pain. They criticize themselves for minor mistakes and strive for perfection to avoid being a burden on anybody.

They also tend to report more physical issues like migraines, chronic pain, autoimmune disorders, or extreme exhaustion. At some point in our sessions, they share their anger around feeling emotionally neglected by those who were supposed to protect them. They mourn for the younger version of themselves who received so much praise for maturity and self-sufficiency instead of getting the care and attention they needed.

Then I see this cycle begin again with the young women I work with who feel pressure to shoulder their families' emotional needs, or worse, to not have any problems at all, fearing it would burden their parents. I've observed it with my college students, especially those who are first-generation or carry significant responsibilities in their families, like translating, contributing to finances, or caring for their younger siblings.

While contributing or showing up for the family can be expected or necessary, the burden of believing you are the primary support for the family when you are young takes a toll on mental well-being. This leaves our girls feeling as though they must prioritize everyone else's needs over their own and thinking they must sacrifice themselves for the greater good, something they will eventually need to unravel as they move through adulthood.

During adolescence, it's more important and developmentally appropriate for girls to be more attuned to what their peers are doing and what they need to develop in alignment with their culture and age group. We still serve as a necessary support and guidance system, but the validation our girls seek will primarily be from peers whom they want to get close to or emulate.

My Interests May Be Different Than Yours; That's Okay

Girls get frustrated when they don't feel like they have room to figure out their interests or believe that they must follow an old pattern rather than carve out their own path. As parents, we dream of our girls doing the things we did, like getting involved in dance, swimming, or soccer, because those activities made our lives meaningful. While it can be enjoyable to introduce our girls to our passions, we also want to make sure we aren't imposing our interests on them and expecting them to follow our footsteps or live our dreams.

There are so many ways our girls can stay active and be fulfilled, and their ability to find these things depends on our willingness to give them space to explore. If we've already decided on or believe we've figured out their path, they may just give in to following what worked in our lives instead of discovering what works for them. This limits their ability to tap into their own intuition or insight to figure out what truly makes them feel like themselves.

I work with many girls who have no idea what they like; they don't even know their favorite color or food. They have difficulty thinking for themselves and instead consider what they think I want to hear when we talk. Their intuitive muscle isn't gone, but it's severely atrophied because it hasn't been exercised enough. They have figured out ways of living that ensure everyone else likes what they do instead of them liking what they do.

One family I worked with enrolled their daughter in dance early, expecting her to continue and compete. This girl injured herself many times and had surgery by the time she was thirteen. When I talked with her about the joy of dancing, she had no idea what I was talking about. She said she didn't experience joy; what she experienced was acceptance—by her family and society. She felt like she was doing what she was supposed to do, specifically what girls typically do, following her family's expectations and what supposedly constituted success for girls in a high school setting.

What she really found joy in was taking pictures and talking about comedy; she even wanted to try comedy herself, but she didn't know where to start. Her parents told her they didn't understand photography, couldn't afford a camera, and didn't see her as naturally funny. She was frustrated because her parents always spent money on dance outfits or competitions, yet she knew a camera would cost much less than the outfits purchased in a year. She knew they wanted her to focus on dancing and were not interested in exploring anything outside of that box.

She took pictures with her phone and had a Finsta account (a fake Instagram account, sometimes called a spam account) to share her pictures of sunsets and animals. She watched her favorite comedians on YouTube and once drove into Chicago with some friends to see a Second City performance. Her parents knew nothing about these experiences, and she knew she couldn't tell them.

This created a significant distance between them, making dance feel like a chore and her parents like a burden, or people she had to pacify. According to her, she was trying to "get through" the time so she could "become herself" after high school. The fact that she, and so many girls I know, are waiting to become themselves once they get out of the home is such a loss for them, but more so a loss for their parents. The inability to hear our girls creates an imbalanced relationship, where we're unwilling to truly understand them, instead favoring our comfort by expecting them to conform to our expectations.

It's yet again something our girls will need to unwind in adulthood, and the women I talk to who feel distant from their adult daughters have difficulty understanding why their daughters wouldn't be grateful to them, rather than frustrated. They believe they helped their daughters achieve success and have difficulty understanding that true success is less about trophies and more about feeling like you are following your passions and doing what feels like you inside.

One of my friends' daughters approached her during her junior year of high school and expressed that she was considering not playing soccer anymore. This girl had been playing since she was very young and had finally reached the varsity level. Instead of my friend telling her daughter about how hard she had worked to get to that point or worrying about what she would do instead, she asked her daughter to put her hand on her heart, take a deep breath, and ask herself if she was truly done with soccer. Her daughter did this and confidently said, "Yes, for sure." And that was that.

She continued to enjoy high school, tried new things, and eventually went to college to become a nurse. Now working a hectic ER schedule, she knows how to prioritize herself and ask for what she needs. Most importantly, she has a trusting and connected relationship with her parents.

There are no guarantees that everything will unfold exactly like this story, and there are no assurances that our girls' passions will align with society's version of success. But what girls do need is a consistent countercultural message about their inherent worth and significance. They shouldn't feel pushed into a toxic achievement culture where everything revolves around seeking external validation and financial reward. What they need to know is that we support their passions and encourage them to pursue what they love. By doing so, they will be more internally motivated, persistent, and resilient. At the very least, they will have hobbies that keep them engaged and content.

One of the most rewarding activities I do with groups of girls in workshops and with my college students is prompting them to reflect on their childhood passions. I encourage them to write about what they genuinely loved and what captured their attention when they were very little. This exercise guides them back to what brought them joy before societal expectations and achievement influences took over.

Sometimes, during these reflections, they rediscover long-forgotten interests and reconnect with experiences that once made them feel like themselves. Our ability to trust what our girls love and focus on what brings them joy not only sets them free to pursue what they enjoy, but also allows them to strengthen their intuitive and instinctual muscles. This helps develop a strong sense of self they will need as they move through college and young adulthood.

Be Curious about What I Know and Love

Girls can feel frustrated when their parents judge, ignore, or disregard the things they love. Much of what our girls love might not make sense to us, but that doesn't mean it doesn't make sense to them. Our girls have different interests because they're from a different generation, and there are different issues in play. With new advances in technology, changes in the celebrity and influencer landscape and whatever they are being exposed to on social media means they're interested in things we may not relate to or fully understand.

Too often, we are much more invested in getting them to like our stuff, our favorite movies and music, our favorite pro teams, our college, our lives. When they aren't interested, we might feel disappointed, because we hoped to bond over these interests. It might lead to questioning whether we're effectively communicating or whether our interests are relevant to them. We might feel a sense of loss, as we had imagined sharing these experiences with them.

But we can also connect by taking an interest in our daughters' interests, allowing them to appreciate our curiosity while also teaching us about themselves, creating a more mutually respectful relationship. It gives us the opportunity to recognize their skills in certain areas and how much they know and can do—whether it's about the music they listen to, their fashion choices, or their hobbies, what they love usually has thought and purpose behind it.

My daughters have taught me so much about the social media influencers they follow, the Gen Z slang they use, the tutorials about clothes, makeup, and even learning how to fix, create, or cook things from YouTube tutorials. They've been able to share clips from their favorite actors, make me a playlist of their favorite songs, and since they were very little, we have always had Taylor Swift.

My girls have loved Taylor Swift since we watched her perform "Mean" at the Grammys in 2012. Since then, they have been experts in her music, business savvy, and life, and their continued interest has kept my husband and me just as consumed. We have loved her through the good and the bad, and for those who get it, our favorite album is still *Reputation*.

Our girls have done podcasts with us about her music, we've attended every concert together since the Red Tour (and we experienced the Eras tour twice), and every album release is a buildup of excitement, staying up late to listen, and then deep conversations for days (years?) about the interpretation of lyrics. Our girls' interest became our interest, and it's developed a way of understanding each other through a decade of music.

There have also been things I didn't understand, whether it's been influencers or commentary that felt hyper-skewed and didn't present a balanced view of information. In these situations, I'm eager to stay engaged and remain a voice of reason when it feels like what they are seeing may not be factual or safe. I still try to stay in the student category, asking questions and allowing them to explain what they think.

Usually, on their own, they come back to a place of reason just by processing through their experience. The reason our kids tend to double down, not listen, or push us away is that we approach them with judgment, making them feel forced to defend their position. But if we can be calm and curious, they are typically open to sharing what they know, and are much more likely to listen when we share our perspective.

CONNECT WITH ME

Feeling Judged by You Makes Me Want to Not Tell You Things

Girls often feel worse after confiding in their parents, especially when it comes to issues regarding friendship or social media. Two of the most common concerns I hear from parents are, "Why doesn't my daughter talk to me about things?" and "How do I get my daughter to share with me?" Our focus should be less on them, and more on how we respond when they do share.

Our daughters don't feel comfortable coming to us about social media issues because our responses tend to include restrictions, blame, or outright forbidding them from using their phones or apps. It's scary for them to lose their social lives and comfort tools all at once, especially when all they're trying to do is engage better and avoid what feels unsafe or uncomfortable. Girls worry about losing all the good parts of social media because of one bad experience, so they end up avoiding talking to us and handling the issue on their own.

Girls also feel particularly judged when it comes to issues with romantic relationships or friendships. We often underestimate the importance or constant presence of these relationships in our girls' lives, and too quickly advise them to break up, sever ties, not tolerate certain behaviors, or simply walk away.

These actions, which might seem like good advice, can sometimes ignore the possible outcomes for our children if they follow them. When we urge them to confront someone or to walk away from a situation, we overlook the confined environment of their world in middle school, high school, or college, where they interact with the same people day in and day out. This means they often need to learn how to manage a situation rather than escalate it.

We also have to consider whether we apply this same advice in our own workplaces or social circle. It's simple to emphasize the importance of doing the "right thing" to our daughters, but are we actively upholding these principles ourselves, or are we holding our girls to a higher standard? And if they do decide to sever ties or not tolerate behaviors, do we provide them with the support they may need to deal with the changes and potential backlash?

We should never suggest that our girls stay in an abusive situation (see Cult and High-Control Group section on page 70); these are times when it's clear they should leave and never look back. But there are other rifts, disagreements, and discomforts that require a more nuanced approach, a way of seeing something differently or relating to it differently rather than disconnecting completely.

RESTORING OUR GIRLS

I recently worked with a girl who was constantly frustrated with someone in her friend group. She found this person annoying in almost every situation and wanted to figure out how to either push this girl out of the group or turn others against her. We explored a lot of options, but most of our discussion centered on how this friend's presence affected her and why she didn't want her around.

She was able to share that she envied the girl because she was talented and socialized easily. We talked about why it's okay to feel envy and how it can show us what we value or desire for ourselves. We worked to reduce any shame she felt about being envious and turn it into something more helpful and clarifying.

We also brainstormed ways for her to distance herself when the feelings became overwhelming, such as journaling about her frustrations or expressing them through artwork. The goal was for her to understand that it's normal to feel annoyed or frustrated with someone, but it's important not to harm others. We emphasized the need to take care of herself when things become too much, while also learning to process uncomfortable feelings and recognizing that situations can change quickly. The last time we talked, she mentioned that the girl now hangs out with a different group, so it's no longer an issue for her.

When our girls tell us they didn't have a partner in gym class, or had nobody to sit with at lunch, they pick up on our reactions. Sometimes, we focus on what they could do differently or how they can become more likable, reinforcing their fear that something is indeed wrong with them. Instead, we can just say "I get it" or "That's rough" without trying to problem-solve. If we can simply relate to their experiences, and maybe even find a way to both laugh, it can help ease the worry and remind our girls that everyone faces challenging social situations.

REAL THINGS GIRLS WANT YOU TO KNOW

We set the tone for how other people react to our children and how our children perceive themselves. If we engage in judgment or gossip, or consistently share negative narratives about our daughter—whether it's something serious, like her mental health, or something more minor, like her taste in clothes—it inadvertently grants permission for others to do or believe the same.

We also don't need to walk around telling everybody how great our daughter is in a bragging way; instead, we simply treat our girls the way we treat others: with dignity and grace. While we may naturally be inclined to share our daughters' successes, we also need to be mindful of how it affects them—whether what we share boosts their confidence and makes them feel seen, or somehow feels like an overshare, leaving them embarrassed.

With good intentions, we can easily get caught up in minor concerns like their dress choice for a dance, focusing on things like its length or fit. This can take away from what we really want for our girls—enjoying themselves, building friendships, and growing up. Some kids end up facing criticisms about their clothing choices in social media comments, or even directly from family members.

I asked Michelle Icard, author of *Eight Setbacks That Can Make a Child a Success: What to Do and What to Say to Turn "Failures" into Character-Building Moments*, about her experience with talking to parents about this, and I love what she had to say:

> Many of us are afraid that our daughter's clothing will attract unwanted attention or harassment. But addressing that fear by asking our girls to dress differently isn't a real form of protection. After all, women and girls face harassment regardless of what they are wearing—even in the most covered, modest outfits.

Instead of saying, "You need to change into something less sexy before you go out," try saying something like this: "Wow, you look great! You look so great you'll probably get a lot of attention, some nice, some potentially uncomfortable. If someone makes you uncomfortable, do you have a plan for how you'll react? Does that plan change if it's someone your age or someone older, or someone in a position of authority?"

Instead of planting seeds of shame, this approach empowers girls to move through the world with confidence.

When You Think of Me, I Feel Less Alone

Girls need to separate from us, and they don't want to feel guilty for doing so. Sometimes they need us for intense or difficult times for a year, a few months, or even a day or two, and hopefully we are willing to show up intensely and then ease up when they are ready to be independent again. This is the dynamic of relationship as our girls get older—showing up when they need us, backing up when they are ready to move forward.

Girls experience their first individuation around age three, when they assert their independence with phrases like "I do it myself!" or emphatic "No!" This marks their readiness to learn through hands-on experience, and it's crucial to give them the space to do so. Around age thirteen, girls undergo another individuation phase, where they may prefer to be dropped off farther from school, go to movies without parental presence, or make their own choices about clothing and hairstyles. This signals their desire to navigate life on their own terms, a process that continues into adulthood. While this transition can be unsettling for parents, it's a natural and necessary part of their development. Understanding and supporting, rather than imposing guilt, keeps the relationship intact.

Space is what they need, but it doesn't mean we should give up or distance ourselves. Instead, we find new ways to connect, reminding them that we understand they are growing up while reassuring them that we're always here. Letting them know we're around and thinking of them reduces their sense of isolation and strengthens the invisible bond between us that they can rely on.

If we feel hurt by their preference to spend time with friends or alone rather than with us, it's easy to react passively or assume that they're being disrespectful or owe us something. While it's important to create a friendly relationship with our girls and treat them more like peers as they mature, we shouldn't expect a friendship where they owe us their time, or a certain level of interaction typically found with adults.

We can have basic expectations, such as having dinner together, family outings, vacations, completing tasks around the house, and respecting curfew. But expecting them to spend as much time with us as they did when they were younger is not realistic.

At the same time, our daughters may go through phases where they experience friend troubles, breakups, or other life challenges, and they may appreciate spending more time at home. This is normal and to be expected; sometimes they need to shut out the world's expectations for a while to regain balance.

Do your best to allow them this time without making them feel guilty or suggesting they need more friends. The better you understand their current situation, the more stability and trust they will have to eventually reengage and put themselves out there again.

Our relationship with our girls is not evenly reciprocal—they will always need more from us than we should expect from them, especially during the teen years, when they are asserting independence but still checking to see if we are there. It's like when our three-year-old starts venturing out and keeps looking back to make sure that we're watching and nearby. They don't necessarily need help (unless they fall and cry), but they also don't want to be left alone.

We can keep in touch with our girls by texting them to just check in, sending them memes, leaving Post-its on their door, or grabbing a quick dinner together when they're free. These acts of love should be genuine, not driven by neediness or manipulation, but as gentle reminders of affection throughout their day. Letting them know we are there isn't about seeking validation or thanks; it's about reassuring them that we're steadfast as they move forward in life.

Rachel Simmons, author of *The Curse of the Good Girl*, spoke at our 2020 Zen Parenting Conference, and I remember her telling the audience that when we provide support or love to our girls, they will rarely, if ever, conclude the interaction with effusive thanks and deep appreciation. We shouldn't expect our girls, particularly teens and young adults, to shower us with gratitude after we've assisted them. Not because they lack kindness, but because they often see our relationship as a dependable anchor, not something they need to reaffirm through praise and compliments.

We are someone they shouldn't fear losing. Certainly, we can teach them about boundaries regarding respect and mutual consideration, such as reminding them to text when they travel or arrive home, because we worry and it's not fair to cause unnecessary concern. However, our relationship shouldn't be conditional or something that they must earn; it should be solid, evolving, adaptable, and understanding.

One night, my daughter was walking with a friend, and I texted her to ask what time she would be home. She responded, and I gave it a thumbs-up. Later, she told me that her friend had mentioned that no one ever checks in with her or asks where she's going, and if she receives a text from her family, it's usually bad news or someone who's upset with her.

As I've said many times, there's a delicate balance here: keeping in touch with our girls without smothering them, allowing them to be independent while ensuring they know we're available. It's a practice that requires ongoing, real conversations to navigate and understand the space they need, or a closeness they can feel.

See My Side When I Tell You a Story

When girls share something vulnerable, they feel frustrated if their parents immediately shift focus away from them and onto the others involved. There will be opportunities to discuss compassionate or empathetic approaches to any situation, but those conversations can come later. Initially, we need to prioritize focusing solely on what our daughter is telling us.

We don't have to agree with everything we hear; our first step should be to acknowledge the pain, fear, annoyance, or any other feelings being shared. Sometimes they may have created their own challenge, and other times they may be the victim in the situation. Regardless, the initial response should be to listen and acknowledge their experience. For example, we can say, "I can see this is upsetting you," or "Wow, that sounds like a lot to handle."

If we too quickly jump to resolving issues, pointing out everything they missed or offering our own feelings or judgments, the conversation will quickly end. There will be time for input, but not right away. When our daughter is feeling overwhelmed, possibly flooded by her feelings, she's not capable of receiving feedback. She only needs to release so she can get clear about what to do next. At that point, she may seek our advice.

We may find ourselves concerned about the other people in the story (*You did what to whom?*), but again, the first priority is to listen. You don't need to advocate for everyone involved in the story they are telling. There will be time to focus on others' needs or perspectives, but that should come after your daughter feels heard.

This is important because, if they share their feelings and everything they say is questioned or others are favored, their focus shifts to being seen and understood, or proving their side of the story. Instead of resolving their feelings, their emotions become tangled or intensified. They not only have their original issue, but also feel misunderstood or invalidated, so we are contributing to the problem. This reinforces the belief that we don't understand, and worse, that they are difficult to manage or unlovable.

Imagine your daughter when she was younger, falling off a swing after she was told not to swing, or when she was swinging too long and probably should have offered it to the next kid in line. When they fall off and hurt themselves, the first step is to make sure they are okay, hold them, listen, and soothe. Once they are in a better state, you can talk about what was expected or how they could have done things differently.

This is just as true with older girls. They need to know that when they fall off socially, emotionally, or academically, there is someone who still sees them and has their back. They need to know that we know they are more than what they do; they are loved for who they are, and we can see through their eyes and hold the wider perspective.

Not Every Conversation Has to Be a Lesson

One of the most common things girls tell me is that they hesitate to talk to their parents about anything because every conversation turns into a lesson. They might share their favorite rapper, only to have their parents explain why rap music is bad. They mention a new favorite app, only to get a lecture about the negative aspects of phones. Even when they excitedly talk about making a new friend through text, their parents express concern about the lack of face-to-face interaction.

It feels like everything our girls want to share becomes an opportunity for us to disrupt or criticize instead of simply engage with them. Consider that when our kids share things with us, they might be making what John and Julie Gottman call "bids for connection"—attempts to share something about themselves with someone they love. These bids may be a comment, a question, a story, an invitation, or a request for help.

Recognizing and positively responding to these bids can profoundly impact our relationship with our daughters. According to Gottman, there are typically three ways we react to these bids: turning toward them by engaging in conversation and connecting, turning away from them by ignoring them or being distracted, or turning against them by responding with lectures, criticism, or annoyance.

Ignoring or rejecting these attempts undermines trust over time and can cause our daughters to withdraw emotionally from us. They may learn not to turn to us when they want to connect or share their lives. Responding positively to these gestures shows our girls that we're attentive and genuinely interested in their lives, without always feeling the need to teach a lesson in every conversation.

While we are bound to make mistakes and may not always respond in the best way to our girls, especially when we're busy or distracted, we can use our repair skills to acknowledge what we've missed. Especially if they later inform us that they were trying to connect and we missed it, we can apologize and ask for a do-over or a chance to try again.

If they try to connect with us while we're on a call, rushing out the door, or otherwise preoccupied, we can let them know we're genuinely interested in what they're saying and that we want to give them our full attention when we listen. We can reassure them that, as soon as we're off the call, finished with work, or back home, we'll circle back and focus on listening and responding. The key is to follow through on this commitment and convey our anticipation for the upcoming conversation.

Your Constant Focus on How I Look Makes Me Worry about It Even More

Parents express concerns about prioritizing their daughters' self-esteem and seek guidance on promoting a positive body image, countering negative messages from diet culture, and navigating situations where their daughters feel inadequate or unattractive.

Girls themselves share these worries, especially when they perceive their parents as overly fixated on their appearance, which only heightens their anxiety. Conversations at home about weight, skin problems, or clothing choices can be particularly distressing for our girls, because they long for a safe environment where their appearance isn't constantly scrutinized.

This is not just a parenting problem; it's a cultural problem. It's not something an individual parent can fix, any more than an individual parent can prevent their daughter from ever being hurt. While our guidance is important, it's also important to understand the complexity and challenges our daughters face without projecting our own fears, concerns, or unresolved issues onto them. We can't shield our daughters from harmful messages, but we can create an environment that minimizes the impact of those messages.

First, we can stop endlessly commenting on their appearance. Of course, we will sometimes tell them they look lovely or that their new outfit is awesome; this is normal discussion. But the majority of what we share needs to be more focused on what they do in the world, how they share their feelings, how they are kind to others, how they respond to disappointment, how they take care of themselves emotionally, how funny they are at dinner, and how great it is that they enjoy time alone as much as they enjoy time with people. Feeling beautiful isn't something inherent in human consciousness. If we think back on the earliest memories of our lives, we will find that we usually felt a lot better about ourselves before we had any idea that society expected us to be beautiful.

Our daughters will inevitably encounter the beauty myth and society's obsession with appearance, but we can help immunize them against it by being less focused on it ourselves. Ideally, we've already done our own work to challenge the expectations for what women should look like and done some healing around our own appearance. But of course, we are all works in progress when it comes to navigating cultural traps and expectations, so we can strive to not exacerbate our daughters' issues by constantly expressing dissatisfaction with our own weight, clothes, wrinkles, or any other aspect of ourselves that we feel doesn't conform to the beauty standard.

When my girls were young and we'd come across magazines while waiting in line at the grocery store, I used the time to explain to them how Photoshop works. I'd tell them how the women on the covers may appear flawless, but it's because their photos have been digitally altered by computers. This helped them understand that the images they see aren't always realistic representations of people.

As they've gotten older, this conversation has continued as social media and filters have taken over. Now my girls know more than I do about why people look the way they do in their pictures, and they explain to me how technology changes appearance, including the fact that people take hundreds of selfies before they post the one that looks so effortless.

We have to keep these discussions going and not add to the problem by criticizing our girls' appearance in photos or comparing them to others (things girls tell me their parents do). This includes commenting on their outfit before school, suggesting they cut or grow their hair, or implying they should eat less because they're gaining weight (things girls tell me their parents say). They already face enough pressure from their peers, the media, and diet culture, and adding our voices only makes them feel more alone and less confident.

Instead, we can help our girls identify with qualities like compassion, curiosity, and hard work, rather than solely focusing on their attractiveness. I've had middle-aged clients and friends who've been consistently praised for their appearance throughout their lives, which shaped their identities around being "pretty." Now, as they get older, they're doing what they can to dismantle this identity because they can no longer rely on their looks.

While beauty played a role in their careers and provided certain privileges, aging has prompted them to pay more attention to different aspects of themselves and to recognize their different values and talents. Many of them have already grown accustomed to cosmetic procedures such as fillers, Botox, and surgeries to maintain a youthful appearance, and would like to be less dependent on altering their looks for approval.

Yes, as women, we get to decide what to do with our faces and bodies, and we don't need to judge women for the choices they make. Every woman gets to choose, and whatever makes them feel more confident or more like themselves should be supported. But most of the time, these women are coming to see me because they are trying to unwind this thinking; they are trying to find more than just appearance to focus their attention on. They are also trying to raise daughters to feel good about themselves, and they know that their lifelong obsession with appearance is being absorbed by their girls—not always by the words they use, but by the actions their daughters see them take.

Their daughters internalize what they see around them, blending societal messages, social media content, what their friends are doing, and most importantly, what their parents are focused on. We either add to the impossible expectations of the culture or we provide a welcome relief and sanctuary from the pressures of the outside world.

In an appearance-obsessed society, we know that people think appearance is important, and negative comments about a person's appearance can be especially hurtful. People who comment negatively or sexually on our daughter's appearance are harming them. Do not excuse this kind of behavior or dismiss it, especially if it is from other family members or close acquaintances. Our daughters need to know that we are on their side, and that their well-being matters more to us than convenience or just trying to maintain the peace.

There have been times when my own daughters have received comments from family members or even strangers, something disparaging, overtly sexual, or just uncomfortable in some way, and I have had to say something like "That's not okay" or "Don't say that" and stop the conversation in its tracks. My goal is to make sure my girls know that they don't need to digest what has been said, that they can leave the comment right there and not pick it up, and that I am willing to disrupt and negate these comments, so they don't have to deal with them alone.

After an experience like this, I've followed up with conversations about what happened, why I intervened, and how they are feeling now. It's always a paradoxical conversation: teaching them that they are not defined by their appearance, while also acknowledging the hurt caused by comments about their appearance. This complexity emphasizes the need to approach these issues from various angles, avoiding simplistic statements like, "You know looks aren't important, so why let it bother you?" which can come across as shaming rather than supportive.

We need to hold space for both truths—recognizing that our girls are much more than their looks, while also acknowledging the societal pressure placed on them about their appearance. Cultural shifts begin when we engage more frequently in these conversations with our daughters and work on ourselves to redefine our own sense of value and worth. By modeling the behavior we want to see and speaking the words we wish to hear, we pave the way for a new perspective on beauty and self-worth.

SUPPORT ME

Even If It Seems Simple to You, I'm Still Learning

Girls feel embarrassed and deeply misunderstood when their parents mock or shame them for not knowing something they believe they should. They get especially irritated when their parents suggest that being young is easy, or that they should be having more fun and not taking things so seriously. All these comments create a major divide, making it obvious that we don't understand our daughters' viewpoint because we're wearing our "adult glasses."

Wearing adult glasses means viewing the world solely through our own eyes and experiences, without attempting to remember what it felt like to be their age. Not a romanticized version of their age, but how it actually feels to experience the pressure of school, social life, extracurricular activities, and an impending future all at once.

When our daughters make poor choices, struggle to regulate their emotions, or even fall apart, we tend to default to criticism or interrogation instead of acknowledging that they're going through a tough time. With their limited life experience and perspective, what they really need from us is compassion and reassurance—a capacity to empathize with their feelings while maintaining our own stability so we can be supportive.

Our girls are not supposed to understand adult pressures because they're not adults. Their experiences and challenges are specific to their age and should be acknowledged as such. Because they haven't lived through the same experiences as us, it's unfair to expect them to react or handle situations as adults would. We shouldn't compare their experiences to ours or expect them to understand adult responsibilities like paying all the bills. This stage of their lives isn't about shouldering those expectations; it's about growth and learning.

It's our responsibility to put on our "teen glasses" again and acknowledge how overwhelming and unpredictable life can feel for our daughters. One of my favorite *Modern Family* episodes is when Claire, the mom, attends a school open house for her daughter Alex, who had an emotional breakdown earlier in the day due to feeling so much pressure. During the open house, Claire realizes how overwhelming the expectations are on Alex and how highly competitive everything is at her school. When Claire comes home and tells Alex how intense it was and how she had no idea of the type of pressure she was under, Alex just hugs her and cries.

The reason our girls choose not to share with us is because they fear being blamed for their overwhelm. Statements like *You shouldn't have taken two AP classes then*, or *You shouldn't hang out with those girls* make them feel worse and ashamed. All they need is for us to get it and to be attentive listeners. To recognize why life feels difficult for them, and to relate. Recognizing that our girls are overwhelmed, rather than debating whether they should be, creates a space for them to talk to us about what feels like too much.

Don't Make Me Feel Guilty for Wanting to Feel Special

There's actual data supporting the benefit of feeling special and knowing we matter. Researchers define "mattering" as the feeling of being a significant part of the world around us, being noticed, important, and needed, and studies show that mattering increases our self-worth and motivation.

Feeling significant also boosts our serotonin levels, which can improve mood and reduce anxiety, and it also reinforces our sense of contribution and purpose, which is associated with what's called the "happiness trifecta" of dopamine, serotonin, and oxytocin, which regulate our mood, movement, and motivation.

As parents, we need to take the lead in reminding our girls why they are special and why they matter. Many women my age were raised in families where shining too brightly was discouraged, often seen as showing off, so they were encouraged to make themselves smaller to avoid burdening others. Unfortunately, some continue to pass this mindset on to their daughters.

As Chimamanda Ngozi Adichie states in *We Should All Be Feminists*, "We teach girls to shrink themselves, to make themselves smaller. We say to girls, you can have ambition, but not too much. You should aim to be successful, but not too successful." We impose limitations on allowing girls to shine, maybe unconsciously to keep them safe or not be threatening to men, but certainly in a way that encourages them to stay small rather than show up fully.

Supporting our girls and celebrating their uniqueness doesn't mean elevating them above others or telling them they are better than other people. Asserting that they're more special than others is untrue and only reinforces unhealthy competition or the pressure to prove superiority. It's about appreciating their strengths and talents while also recognizing those of others. Each of us has something unique to offer, and by embracing our individuality, we help them understand that there isn't just one spotlight to compete for.

We can celebrate our daughters' successes by directly sharing our praise with them, rather than oversharing on social media or boasting to others. Girls have told me how their parents don't communicate with them directly, but they stumble upon lengthy posts written solely about them on social media, maybe for a birthday or graduation. While they appreciate the acknowledgment, they describe feeling disconnected, as if their parents prioritize sharing praise with strangers rather than communicating it directly to them.

Over the years, I've seen how the need for validation shows up in different ways—like seeking attention through relationships, focusing too much on looks, or trying to embody what Gen Z describes as a "pick-me" girl. This refers to someone who prioritizes male approval over friendships with other girls, sometimes distancing themselves from typical girl activities to emphasize their uniqueness.

These girls strive to appear cool to guys, occasionally being unkind to other girls to gain attention. It highlights the immense pressure on girls to seek validation from guys and their desire to feel distinct and separate from the crowd.

While affirming our girls' significance and recognizing their uniqueness at home may not eliminate all "pick-me" tendencies, since seeking attention is natural, especially in our teen years, providing validation at home can certainly reduce the need to devalue others to assert our own specialness.

Please Understand My Fear of Disappointing Others

Most of us know that FOMO is the fear of missing out, but a group of girls were just telling me they have just as much FODO, the fear of disappointing others. They find themselves caught between what they want and the expectations placed on them by family, friends, and society. They experience a lot of pressure, and the fear of disappointing ranks pretty high on their list of their concerns.

It's understandable that, for young girls, validation and recognition from others carry significant weight, and the fear of disappointing anyone stems from the belief that they must meet, and even exceed, the standards set by those around them to be worthy. The pressure to conform to various expectations—whether it's excelling academically for their parents, fitting in with friends, or adhering to societal norms—feels like a full-time job.

The fear of disappointment often triggers feelings of inadequacy and self-doubt because girls compare themselves to others, believing they need to attain impossible standards to succeed in life. One of my daughter's closest friends described it as "swimming against a rip current that fluctuates in strength, regardless of how hard I strive to get it all right."

Girls may say they are doing just fine, but deep down, they're worrying about whether they are doing it "right." We can, and should, remind them, repeatedly, that mistakes and challenges are to be expected as they grow and learn, and that perfection doesn't exist. They need to know that at home, they have the space to discover and develop their true selves without feeling the pressure to meet impossible standards.

How we manage situations at home greatly impacts our daughters' perceptions and interactions with the world. Our expectations develop their understanding of acceptance, and if we convey that mistakes are unacceptable or devalue them when they happen, they enter every other situation fearing they'll make mistakes and won't be loved.

Instead of constantly pushing our girls to achieve and excel, we can redirect our focus to their effort, embracing what researcher Carol Dweck calls a "growth mindset." This mindset acknowledges that skills and talents can be developed through hard work, in contrast to a fixed mindset which implies that abilities are innate—you either have them or you don't. By adopting a growth mindset at home, our daughters can shift their focus from believing they need to perform perfectly to instead focusing on the experience of learning and growing and trusting themselves to do so.

We can support this process by helping our girls establish boundaries when it comes to school or social pressures. But before that, we need to ensure we understand the definition of boundaries ourselves. Social media introduces people to mental health and psychological terms, but it's not always accurate and lacks the necessary context and nuance. Boundaries are not meant to be a form of control or a way to demand things from others, like "My boundary is that you don't spend time with people I don't like" or "My boundary is that we only eat where I want to eat."

Boundaries are personal guidelines that help us determine what's acceptable and what's not in every situation, so we know when to speak up, bow out, or even join in based on what feels right to us. Some examples include expressing when alone time is needed or when a topic of conversation is uncomfortable, asking for consent before hugging someone, setting limits on socializing with toxic or draining people, and prioritizing relationships that are supportive and enriching.

Learning to set and maintain boundaries helps our daughters prioritize themselves within their social and romantic relationships and achieve academically, without overextending themselves to the point of illness, self-neglect, or losing sight of what's most important.

By helping them prioritize their own needs, we reduce the likelihood that they will equate their worth solely with productivity and their contributions to others. Many older women I work with are currently dealing with the harmful messaging ingrained in them about the fear of disappointing others. Unfortunately, it often takes illness, the loss of a marriage, or financial struggles for them to realize they no longer wish to live under this scrutiny and that change is necessary.

Ask Me Before You Post about Me on Social Media

One of the simplest things we can do is ask our girls for permission before sharing their image on social media for everyone to see and comment on. Seeking their consent before sharing a photo is another type of boundary, demonstrating that we respect their wishes and acknowledge their right to decline.

Our girls need to know that their image belongs to them, and they don't have to share it unless they feel comfortable doing so. By demonstrating consideration and modeling respect for their privacy, we encourage them to extend the same courtesy to all the people in their lives.

Our girls are dealing with their own insecurities, especially during the teenage years, and sharing a picture of them, especially if they don't like it or think it's good, can magnify these feelings and make them feel vulnerable or that we don't have their best interest in mind.

From our perspective, we need to consider who will see the picture and why we're sharing it. Often, consciously or unconsciously, we post pictures and write captions that showcase our children's achievements to boost our own ego or impress others. Our girls are quite aware of this, and many find it annoying. One girl described it as "feeling like a prop being used for attention."

When I ask them how to address this, the solution is simple—they just want their parents to ask them first. Sometimes it's no big deal, and they're okay with their parents sharing pictures of vacations or special events, but they want to be considered before their image and lives are posted for the world to see.

Help Me Work through This Grief

> **Trigger warning:**
> There is discussion of gun violence, suicide,
> and suicidal ideation in this section.

There's a significant amount of grief in this generation, and it's unclear whether it's because we understand grief better and can articulate and share it, or if there's simply more to grieve.

What I've observed is that girls experience profound sadness and struggle to understand or cope with it. Our culture's handling of grief is lacking, viewing it as something to bypass or bulldoze through, rather than process. This means families often avoid addressing or discussing it, usually because we, the adults, are dealing with our own grief. If we weren't given space to deal with it, we don't have enough space to help our girls deal with theirs.

Grieving is the most natural and necessary response to loss. It's uncomfortable, but it is inherently healing and necessary. It's the inability to feel and grieve that can make us sick and stuck. Grief involves recognizing both the intense moments of sorrow and how it evolves over time. Contrary to Elizabeth Kübler-Ross's linear model, which pop psychology and social media tend to rely on, grief doesn't progress predictably through stages like denial, depression, and acceptance. Those stages might be felt, but research indicates many diverse trajectories of grief, challenging the idea of some kind of fixed or predictable process.

Clinical psychologist Mary-Frances O'Connor, author of *The Grieving Brain*, emphasizes grief as a universal experience in which connecting and sharing with others allows us to feel better and regain trust. She considers grief a form of neurological learning, where our brains are trying to integrate our new reality while figuring out how to interact with the world in a new way. Grieving takes time, and as author Nora McInerny so profoundly shared, "We don't move on from grief; we move forward with it."

When our girls are young and grieving, it's an essential time to be available to them as their brains learn to reprocess the world. It doesn't mean they will talk to us about every stage and feeling, but we can be available for these real conversations and accept, or at least understand, the volatility of emotions. We shouldn't impose a timetable or expectation on their grief, nor should we make them feel guilty or ashamed for discussing certain aspects of loss repeatedly. They need space without judgment, and the more they have, the better they will understand themselves and process their pain.

Feeling grief is like being hit by a wave and having the wind knocked out of us. Then we practice standing up in the chaos, taking another breath so we can keep going, and possibly getting hit by another wave. Grief is feeling at the deepest, most raw level. It's not the same as depression, which usually involves hopelessness or an inability to feel. Instead, it's us in our most sensitive state, when every nerve is hyper-aware.

Our girls need to understand grief so they're less afraid of it when they feel it. They should know that feeling tired, forgetful, losing their appetite (or gaining one), wanting to be alone or to never be alone are all normal ways of grieving—things they don't need to be afraid of or try to stop.

Our family has made a practice of putting grief and loss out in the open, with plenty of space to be seen and discussed. When our girls were young and our first fish and pet rabbit died, we had our first outdoor ceremony and sharing of feelings. We left the bowl out and the cage up to remember and allow us to process rather than avoid or move on too quickly. Then we could feel it for awhile, until we all agreed it felt like time to put their things away and replace them with pictures and drawings.

When the girls were young and Todd's mom died quite suddenly, we put pictures of her everywhere, talked about every memory, discussed why it felt unfair for her to die so young, and processed how scary it can be to have a person there one day and then have her be gone the next. The girls took days off school, we had more long dinners, and we took long walks. We decided that seeing sunflowers meant she was around, and we searched for them on walks or in pictures.

As my girls watched my dad go through congestive heart failure, we talked about the discomfort and his pain, why it was hard to talk about, and how we could continue to support him and make him more comfortable. When he died, we put his pictures everywhere, and we had a brick installed at our local park so we could visit it and remember him.

RESTORING OUR GIRLS

We decided that a deer represented him best, so whenever we see a deer, or many deer, we know Grampa is around.

My dad had been sick for seventeen years before he died, so my girls also watched me go through significant grief after his death. I was sick for over a month, finally processing years of worry and emotional pain (see Somatics and Embodiment section on page 91). I did my best to explain what was happening, to honor the process of what I was going through so my girls didn't have to be scared or wonder.

A few years later, when my mom slowly deteriorated through dementia, we discussed how to talk and relate to her now that she was changing, and how difficult it can be to go through what is called anticipatory grief, which is a slow, continuous process of grieving as we care for someone whose abilities are changing, and adjusting to the loss of their previous self. We talked about the discomfort in seeing her, as well as the joy in seeing her, especially when she remembered things.

When she died, we again put her pictures everywhere, shared stories, and recognized the loss of so many grandparents. We discussed how death can feel like a relief, as well as a kick in the stomach, and how this paradox of mixed emotions is nothing to be ashamed of, but only a reality as we let go of people who we have watched suffer. We decided that she was best represented as a butterfly, so we acknowledge her whenever we see one fly by.

Our daughters will most likely have to grieve adults who die due to age or illness, and sometimes they are grieving friends who die, often tragically, which adds another layer of understanding mortality and their sense of safety. I know too many teen girls who know someone who has died in a shooting of some type, and they see dying by gun violence as a reality of their generation.

They also know kids who have died by suicide, and there is a silence and discomfort in knowing how to proceed or talk about it. Suicide is surrounded by stigma, and we don't want to pass judgment on why or how it happened, or even worse, decide who to blame. Instead, we continue to speak about and use the name of the person who died, share our memories of that person, and honor this person who will be missed. Their life was much more than their death.

If our girls share that they have suicidal thoughts or have made attempts, conversations are often avoided; we talk around the subject instead of addressing it directly. As a clinician, I am well-practiced in openly addressing these questions when the girls and women I work with tell me they are depressed, and I ask if they have thoughts of hurting themselves or taking their lives. If the answer suggests a yes, I keep asking questions to assess whether these are vague thoughts or an actual plan to follow through. For parents these are scary questions, and involving professionals make it easier to know what to do next.

People experiencing suicidal thoughts want their fears and feelings to be heard without judgment, and encouraging open discussion could potentially serve as a preventative measure. When discussing this with parents, some have told me that they advised their depressed and often suicidal daughters not to talk about such things and to keep their struggles hidden. Secrecy only intensifies the burden, and not recognizing this only increases feelings of shame and guilt. There's still a belief that talking about suicide might promote it, but staying silent only makes it harder to cope and perpetuates the stigma surrounding mental health.

Sometimes the grief our girls feel is around more common issues, like changing friend groups or schools, losing a romantic relationship, or simply growing up. They feel the pain of transition and experience feelings of being lost, guilty, or alone, especially when they compare

RESTORING OUR GIRLS

their pain to that of others, which I advise them to not do—in clinical terms, this is called comparative suffering, and it's not helpful because it undermines the validity of our experiences and can prevent us from getting the support we need.

Allowing our girls to speak openly about their sadness and to acknowledge the possible paradox—for example, they are excited to grow up, but they also miss childhood—allows their brains to integrate their new experiences, rather than hide them or be embarrassed by feeling them. It's a way to normalize their feelings and remind them they aren't alone.

As our girls grieve, we can ask open-ended questions that respect their feelings and empower them to control their own narrative:

- "Can you tell me more about what this has been like for you?"
- "Most people have strong feelings when something like this happens. What has this been like for you?"
- "I noticed you did/said ___. I was wondering how you might be feeling."
- "What kinds of memories do you have about (the person who died)?"
- "What will you miss the most about high school?"
- "What sorts of things have you been thinking about since your breakup?"

Reminding them that there are many ways to grieve and just as many ways to heal, I tell the girls I work with to utilize the things they love—writing, drawing, dancing, talking—to navigate through it. I challenge them to honor what they are going through and find ways to express what's inside without expectations, time limits, or concern for how it looks. Sometimes grief is a gentle cry, and sometimes it's a screaming fit. There isn't a right way; it's about trusting our bodies and minds to know what we need.

TRUST ME

~

Guidance Is Great; So Is Making Some Decisions on My Own

Our girls need our support, but they also need us to believe in what they can do themselves. Our ability to stand back and allow them to make decisions on their own—whether it's choosing their classes, their outfits, or their friend group—is necessary for developing the autonomy they need to succeed independently.

Some parents believe that, as long as their children are living under their roof, they have the right to manage every aspect of their lives. But as their daughters enter adolescence, it becomes important, and developmentally appropriate, for them to start taking charge of some of their own decisions.

Parents who struggle to give up control may inadvertently push their daughters toward seriously rebelling. While initially compliant, girls with overly controlling parents often resort to breaking rules and then hiding their choices. Then they distance themselves and avoid seeking help if they end up in trouble, to continue hiding their behavior. This tug-of-war between parents pointing fingers at their daughters for hiding things and the daughters feeling suffocated by their parents' control is a common dynamic I help families untangle.

RESTORING OUR GIRLS

Our daughters aren't meant to follow paths set by us—they're individuals, with their own needs and interests. Empowering our daughters to explore what they love also involves encouraging them to trust their instincts. This requires us to take a step back and allow for pursuits beyond just academic achievements. When we allow our girls the freedom to figure out what really interests them, they will naturally invest more effort and enthusiasm. By loosening our grip and letting them discover what resonates with them, we help them become successful.

Girls are more likely to be self-disciplined and motivated when they feel a strong sense of control over their lives, and research points to *agency* as one of the most significant factors contributing to their success and happiness. Agency predicts the positive outcomes we want for our girls: enhanced health and longevity, decreased substance abuse, reduced stress, heightened emotional well-being, increased intrinsic motivation and self-discipline, improved academic performance, and even greater career achievement.

Every semester my college students share the challenges of their parents' micromanagement. They describe how their parents determine their majors, choose their classes, select their dorms, and even dictate when they should reach out to teachers for assistance. I also hear similar stories from adolescent girls who express interest in specific clubs or sports, only to find their parents have already made decisions for them regarding their extracurricular involvement or which AP classes they'll take.

It's okay, and even necessary, to offer our kids support and guidance, but we need to balance this with allowing them a sense of sovereignty over their choices and lives. One of the most important things we can do when our girls come to us for help is to start with the question, "What do you think?" After considering their needs, then the door is open to offer some guidance and support.

REAL THINGS GIRLS WANT YOU TO KNOW

Don't Compare My Teen Challenges to Your Teen Challenges

We are all very quick to share our stories of high school, to remind our girls that we've gone through what they've gone through and that we totally get what it means to be a teen. Yes, we've been their age, but we've never been their age in our current society, and we've never been their age with their group of friends, their community, their classes, and their teachers.

We may have some understanding or memories of teen angst, but we need to at least consider that our girls are having very different experiences than we did, and that giving them the advice that we latched onto when we were their age may not work in this space and time. This group of young women, born between 1997 and 2012, has grown up in the shadow of social media, climate change fears, and the COVID-19 pandemic, and plenty of experts say they've developed different priorities than older generations. Asking them to do what we did to stay safe or telling them how we had it harder does not lead to connection; it just makes them feel like we don't get it.

A study of 36,000 people around the world, commissioned by the New York-based BCW communications firm, found 43 percent of GenZers actively seek opportunities for fun and prioritize activities that bring them pleasure, a significantly higher percentage than any other generation. They are also more inclined to take gap years and explore alternative educational paths based on their interests or desire to travel.

This doesn't mean they are checked out or don't take life seriously. According to a recent survey by the Pew Research Center in the US, members of Gen Z are the most racially and ethnically diverse generation yet, and they are poised to become the most well-educated. Girls from this group have ambitious life goals and engage in thoughtful discussions about things like entrepreneurship, addressing climate change, and using their platforms and voices to create political change.

We can share our stories, but we should remember they may not directly apply to our daughters' experiences, nor should we expect them to follow our exact path. For instance, while volleyball might have been popular when we were in school, it may not hold the same appeal in theirs. Similarly, finding a job or volunteer position may have been easier in our youth than in today's competitive environment. It's about shifting our perspective, taking off our "adult glasses," and seeing their world through their eyes.

Let Me Hold onto Things from My Childhood

Our home has so many streaming services, and when it came time to make some cuts, both my teenage and adult daughters were adamant about keeping Disney+. When I asked why it was so important to them, they explained that Disney+ carries all their beloved childhood movies, serving as a source of comfort and nostalgia when they need to unwind.

My daughters still have stuffed animals that live on their beds, and their friends from college also have stuffed animals or special blankets that live on their beds in their dorm rooms. When our girls were little, these items could be called transitional objects, a concept introduced by psychoanalyst Donald Winnicott that refers to a specific object, usually a toy or blanket, that a child uses as a source of comfort during times of stress or anxiety, especially when separated from their primary caregiver.

Transitional objects serve as a bridge between a child's inner world and their external reality, providing a sense of security and familiarity that helps them cope with the challenges of growing autonomy and independence. These objects play an important role in early childhood development and continue to hold symbolic importance for our girls as they navigate the transition from dependence to autonomy.

The truth is the transition from dependence to autonomy is a work in progress from adolescence to post-college, and allowing our girls to have whatever they need to make this process less daunting is important. When we make fun of what makes our girls feel comforted, or tell them they've outgrown the things they love, we are taking away their coping mechanisms and asking them to let go of sources of security.

It's an antiquated belief that we outgrow the things that brought us comfort in childhood. Even as adults, it's important to keep playing, channeling our imagination, and practicing our creativity if we want to have a meaningful and fulfilling life. Research demonstrates the significance of continuing to play and embracing a childlike mindset as we age. Dr. Stuart Brown, head of a nonprofit called the National Institute for Play, emphasizes the necessity and meaning of play for adults, saying, "Play is something done for its own sake. It's voluntary, pleasurable, offers a sense of engagement, takes you out of time, and the act itself is more important than the outcome."

Playing and holding onto childlike wonder doesn't imply immaturity; it's about staying open and aware, finding joy in the simple things. Take my own stuffed monkey, for example, that I've had since I was two. He's been with me through college, every apartment, and every home, and now, he sits in a rocking chair in my current bedroom. He's been through it all with me, and I often tell my husband and girls that he knows me better than anyone because he's been there since the very beginning.

If I Push Myself Too Hard, Remind Me That Life's about More than Grades

Ideally, schools can focus on our girls' learning and academics, while we can prioritize their overall well-being. If this balance is disrupted, our girls can easily get confused about what makes them lovable and valuable, and what it means to be smart.

Again, ideally, it's beneficial to encourage your daughter to take ownership of her grades. This can be challenging due to systems like PowerSchool or other web-based student information systems used by school districts. These systems make it too easy to get involved, and sometimes teachers expect us to be involved. But we can easily become overly invested in monitoring every aspect of our daughter's academic performance because we can see everything that's happening. My daughters' friends have told me about receiving texts from their parents in the middle of the school day, asking why they received a C on a test, even though they had just finished the test thirty minutes before.

With so much information readily available, our girls feel constant pressure to excel, and they feel unable to escape because their parents have access to every detail of their academic experience. We can offer support by finding tutors or study materials, or by simply being available for guidance, but being more focused on their academic outcomes then they are will not only push them away from us, but will exert an excessive kind of pressure that makes them lose track of what's most important in life.

Girls I've worked with who have had to tell their parents about their struggles with mental health, eating disorders, substance abuse, self-harm, or suicidal thoughts have helped their parents realize the secondary importance of academic achievement compared to their

REAL THINGS GIRLS WANT YOU TO KNOW

overall well-being. These challenges prompt parents to prioritize their daughters' sense of self, understanding that while academics are important, they pale in comparison to their daughters' health and safety.

This holds true not only in times of crisis, but also when crises aren't apparent. Academic achievement can create a narrow tunnel vision, leading us to believe it's the sole path to our daughters' success, and that every dream and opportunity hinges on it. I've encountered dozens of girls who dedicated themselves tirelessly to high school, barely lifting their heads to prioritize their well-being, all in pursuit of their dream college or career.

Too many of them end up drinking too much once they get to college, failing classes, or completely dropping out because they never learned how to practice self-care or make themselves a priority. Sometimes they return to school after addressing their mental health needs and rediscovering their footing, but this process takes time, and a complete redefining of what success looks and feels like.

Instead of waiting for a crisis or pushing our girls forward without consideration, we can help them in balancing other aspects of their identity and interests alongside their academic goals. If they solely define themselves by grades or test scores, receiving a low grade, even a B, will profoundly affect their self-esteem. In these cases, they might become even more hyper-focused on academic success, or completely give up to avoid pain and disappointment, which could lead them to feel that school or learning isn't for them.

Feeling this pressure doesn't just resolve itself even if they push through and finish college or higher degrees; they usually carry the same unforgiving patterns into the workplace, and even when starting families, lacking the necessary coping mechanisms to handle disappointment or lack of control over outcomes.

RESTORING OUR GIRLS

Many of the moms I work with now were once high achievers in school, and still struggle to tolerate any form of failure, real or perceived. They still feel compelled to maintain a façade of perfection or success, resulting in emotional pain or even physical symptoms and illness. While these patterns can be addressed and unlearned in therapy, why would we perpetuate this pattern and endorse these behaviors in our girls? We know they are unsustainable and harmful in the long run.

We need to remember and remind our girls that there are many forms of intelligence, and that academic achievement, grades, or IQ are just one aspect. Emotional intelligence, for instance, is a much stronger predictor of success in both work and life, yet it often doesn't receive the recognition it deserves in formal education.

When my oldest daughter struggled with school pressure and the belief that others had an easier time with certain classes or expectations, I constantly reminded her to take a wider lens on the word "intelligence." While some of her peers might find multiple-choice tests simple or were able to memorize the periodic table with ease, my daughter excelled in discussing literature, exploring new places, tending to others' emotional well-being, and building connections with people from all walks of life.

We don't need to belittle others' skills or intelligence to appreciate our own. Recognizing the diverse talents and strengths of others not only deepens our empathy and understanding, but also reminds us that people have a range of skills to tackle the complex issues in our world. We aren't all supposed to be good at everything, or even the same things, and this reminds us to pursue what we love. Our brains are wired to excel in areas we're passionate about, and trying to follow someone else's path contradicts our innate inclinations and talents.

REAL THINGS GIRLS WANT YOU TO KNOW

LAUGH WITH ME

~

Can We Be Less Serious and Have More Fun?

Sometimes, it feels like there's this invisible guidebook, dictating that every interaction with our daughters must be serious, instructional, always pointing out flaws, and keeping a watchful eye on every little detail of their lives. But during all this seriousness, we overlook the simple joy of just kicking back, relaxing, and laughing with our girls.

Our daughters need to know that we understand life's absurdities, that not every challenge is a huge deal. Some situations just require some shrugging and laughter and an acknowledgment that things happen, and it's okay to move on. Our daughters want a connection beyond parental authority, where laughter can be normal without the heavy burden of constant scrutiny or judgment. It's disheartening for them when they share a story and immediately sense our need to teach or criticize, rather than simply laugh about life's randomness.

This is true when it comes to sports and other activities, too. Competition can be important and team sports have valuable lessons, but the relentless pressure to always win and excel overshadows the enjoyment of the game. Moving up to higher divisions or travel teams can be motivating at times, but it can also lead to overwhelming stress. These activities, originally meant to bring joy to their lives, shouldn't become burdens that weigh them down, turning their passions into sources of anxiety and added pressure.

Not every girl is striving to be a professional athlete, musician, or whatever else they are practicing. They're simply exploring their interests during middle school, high school, and college, as age-appropriate experimentation. When extracurricular activities demand an all-consuming dedication that leaves little room for simple enjoyment, then they require some examination.

Girls observe how effortlessly parents engage with their friends, neighbors, and other adults. They confide in me about their confusion, noting the stark contrast between the easygoing, cheerful demeanor their parents exhibit outside the home and the more solemn, stressed, and overwhelmed version they encounter within it. They express disappointment that their parents are often unwilling to share their lighter, more relaxed selves with them.

Our girls not only want to enjoy moments with us, but also want to know that prioritizing fun in life is acceptable. Prioritizing busyness and achievement in our daughters' lives can lead us to overlook what contributes to their well-being. While most parents tell me that what they want most is for their daughter to be happy, their actions and expectations convey the message that being overburdened and overwhelmed is normal and acceptable. Sometimes we accept a level of joylessness without realizing it, and we don't recognize the toll it's taking on us and our girls.

We can cast aside the pressures of perfection in parenting, the relentless demands for success, and just share a laugh with our girls about life's craziness. Whether it's bonding over TV shows, going to Starbucks together, or simply exchanging a knowing eyeroll when life gets too lifey, we can demonstrate to our daughters that we hold a clear and protective stance on what matters most.

Think about Being My Age and What You Needed

When I work with moms, we often discuss what they missed out on or needed when they were younger. It could be something as simple as wanting to hear certain words from their parents, having someone advocate for them at school, or just wishing their homes were happier, calmer, or places that felt more like a respite or safe haven.

Mostly, it comes down to feeling safe and seen. They just wanted to hear that they mattered and that their needs were important. When I was young, I remember my dad telling me that, no matter what, he'd always prioritize taking my call if I called him at work. I didn't test it much, usually only in emergencies or when I felt sick at school. But just hearing him say it so many times made me feel safer and more important.

A lot can remain unspoken when we are young. As parents, we figure our kids understand that we've got their backs, and they mean the world to us. But what they usually hear, through words or actions, is how busy we are, how they stress us out, or how they make our lives too difficult. Sometimes they realize we are just overwhelmed or maybe we are just being funny, but if we don't mix in some real reminders that they matter the most to us, they begin believing that they are too much to handle and we don't have the space. That's when they start backing away and asking for way less.

When our daughters are struggling with something, we can empathize with their experiences and reflect on what kind of support would have been helpful to us during hard times. Take, for instance, the nerve-wracking process of learning to drive, when making mistakes while learning was inevitable. How did receiving criticism or harsh words impact our confidence and ability to learn? Did it truly help us grow, or did it exacerbate an already difficult situation? By drawing from our past experiences, we can create a more compassionate and effective approach to being supportive when things are difficult.

If we can't remember our teenage feelings, we can consider similar situations in our current lives. When we forget something important at home or work, is it helpful if our partner or boss scolds us and tells us we are a disappointment? Or is it more helpful when they are understanding and acknowledge that mistakes happen because we're human? It's too easy to think we can speak to our girls with a disrespectful or harsh tone, believing it's what parents do or that it motivates them, but the majority of the time it just makes them feel ashamed rather than smarter.

When my girls are struggling, I often suggest they chat with their aunt, cousin, or friend who has been through something similar. When they are in a more vulnerable state, they are often more willing to seek guidance from someone who understands. As parents, we can help build these bridges by connecting them with people, therapists, or groups that could offer support. Being able to share their experiences with someone who truly understands and has been there can help them move forward. If they end up forming relationships with these people and they become an additional source to depend on or laugh and cry with, it's even more impactful and rewarding.

Let Me Relax

Most of us are comfortable with relaxing, and we often encourage our daughters to do so, but we often have a specific idea of what relaxation should look like, and we set a time limit around how much relaxing should really be done. Instead of considering what our girls need, we consider our comfort level with what they are doing. When this time limit is reached, or relaxation starts to deviate from our definition, the word that starts getting used is lazy. I can't tell you how many parents have told me that their daughter is lazy, that she comes home from school unmotivated, heads to her room or sits around the house.

Most of the time these girls have just been at school for eight hours—they had early morning band or yearbook staff, then a full day of classes, tests, socializing, feeling left out, feeling overwhelmed, making sure they don't offend anybody, making sure their teacher knows they are trying, making sure they are doing things right. Then they come home, hoping to sit on the couch or go to their room—maybe for a whole hour. Doesn't this make sense?

As adults we have forgotten the day-in-day-out of school—yes, we have the day-in-day-out of work and parenting, which is difficult—but the day-in-day-out of school is also exhausting, and it's full of expectation and not a lot of autonomy. Maybe your daughter has a free period, or maybe she gets to leave for lunch, but most of the time it's one thing on top of the next, over and over, every day. They can do it, it's possible, but for them to do it well, they need time and space to rest.

When the adults in the home tell them that sitting around after school is laziness, it only feels disregarding and diminishing. A fifteen-year-old girl I was talking to recently said, "I try so hard. I go to school, I go to practice, I try to be social with my friends and not piss anyone off, I try to like all the things my friends are posting and keep my streaks alive—then I do homework, stay up way too late, try to pay attention to what's happening in the house and do what people are telling me to do, then I start the whole thing over again, every single day."

Plus, lazy fails to capture the many different types of experiences our girls may be having—maybe they're decompressing, seeking to avoid stress, integrating something that was scary and unexpected, taking a necessary breather, contemplating their next steps, or simply daydreaming and allowing their imagination to wander. These activities are not only normal, but also necessary for their well-being.

The obsession with productivity is pervasive in our culture, where our worth gets measured by how much we check off our lists rather than by how we are feeling and managing life. When asked about our well-being, we default to listing everything we have done or still need to do, equating our busyness with our value.

We may have expectations of our daughter that she show up for family dinner or do her laundry. That's understandable, but telling them they are lazy on a regular basis, or creating a family culture where resting isn't necessary or acceptable, gives our girls only a few choices—either they stay constantly busy and burn out, or they completely avoid us so they don't have to hear how they aren't doing enough.

The best option is to discuss with them what's expected at home and then let them choose how they spend their downtime, whether they need a nap, or how they refuel after a long day. We also need to reflect on why we feel so uncomfortable when we see our girls relaxing—what assumptions are we making?

Many of us feel that we must appear constantly busy, fearing that we will be shamed or judged if someone sees us as unproductive. I am not immune to this—sometimes when I'm sitting down at home and I hear a car pull into the driveway, I jump and start cleaning the kitchen or putting things away. I haven't even had time to think about why I am doing this, I almost do it instinctively, like I'm worried someone will "catch" me relaxing. The societal pressure to be "busy," and that busy makes us valuable, is deeply ingrained, leading us to prioritize activity over well-being. If we're caught relaxing, we scramble to justify our inactivity, fearing we will be accused of not being good enough.

This begins with the expectations of a full school day and plenty of after-school activities. We set our kids up to go from one thing to the next, to keep up with what society tells us is important. This pattern, if continued, can lead to burnout and other mental health challenges in high school or college. If it persists into adulthood, it may become a lifelong habit, raising questions about when it will ever stop. Will it take illness, disconnection from themselves or others, or intense anxiety about self-worth? Many women I speak with currently experience these pressures—they keep their calendars full, their work and social lives busy, to avoid slowing down and feeling. This vicious cycle can eventually pose serious health risks.

Research shows that women account for around 80 percent of all autoimmune disorders, like lupus, rheumatoid arthritis, and multiple sclerosis. Women face a higher risk of chronic pain, sleep problems, and conditions like fibromyalgia and irritable bowel syndrome, as well as long COVID and migraines. They're also twice as likely to die after a heart attack. Depression, anxiety, and PTSD affect women at double the rate of men, and they're nine times more likely to have anorexia, the deadliest mental health disorder.

Scientists have suggested probable reasons for this, including differences in hormones, genetics, and exposure to certain environments, but psychosocial factors, like the pressure on women to always be agreeable, never angry, and excessively selfless, also seem to play a role in women's vulnerability to these illnesses. It may be a combination of factors, but one thing that can help in every situation is the ability to take care of ourselves and prioritize rest as necessary, rather than something to avoid or hide.

Enjoy Your Life So I Can Look Forward to Being Your Age

Do you remember when you were young and heard about people who were thirty? They seemed so old, completely out of touch, and we felt like we were light years away from where they were. I remember in my early twenties when I was at a bar and noticed a group in the back room celebrating their thirtieth birthday. I couldn't help but wonder why they were choosing to celebrate in a bar. Hadn't they transitioned to more mature lives by now?

The fact that I celebrated both my thirtieth and fortieth birthdays in a bar is why I remember this experience so well; I had no conception that people continue going out and having fun after a certain age. I also remember my friend asking my sister, who was twenty-one and had just graduated from college, if she still listened to music or if she only listened to talk radio now that she had a job. Now, think about what our girls might feel about turning forty or fifty—it seems ancient to them, so out of touch and difficult to relate to.

When we're young, our concept of adulthood often feels far removed from reality. We have no idea what brings joy or purpose to someone older, and adults can easily come across as awkward and cringey. Some adults actually fit that description, especially if they are at one extreme or the other—either clinging desperately to youth or fully surrendering to old age and cynicism, just going through the motions of life.

Our girls deserve older role models who prioritize getting the best out of life at every age, rather than solely focusing on looking "hot" and staying wrinkle-free at forty-five, which tends to be more about clinging to youth. It's more about embracing life, following our dreams, establishing strong relationships, pursuing interesting hobbies, and leading a joyful life. It's about focusing on utilizing the wisdom gained from living, maintaining a willingness to continue learning, and then sharing that wisdom with others.

I talk with countless women who share how much they love getting older and embracing who they are becoming with age. They feel liberated, more authentic, more empowered to speak their minds, and more connected to their true selves. This is the kind of role-modeling and conversations that our girls need—stories about how womanhood becomes richer and more deeply understood as we grow older. This doesn't diminish the ongoing challenges we face in terms of equality, aging, and other life challenges, but it offers a nuanced perspective, showing that there's plenty more to look forward to and appreciate as we move through life.

Our girls love getting to know us better and learning to appreciate what we love. My daughters see me enjoying everything from the Backstreet Boys and Greta Van Fleet to Tim McGraw and Yacht Rock, along with '80s hair bands, Taylor Swift, and most classic rock. They see me attending these concerts, dressing up for Halloween, playing my drums, and hosting my own birthday parties. They know I love podcasting and writing, and that I love speaking in front of groups and teaching classes.

They know there's plenty I don't like to do. I'm not the biggest fan of board games, long-distance travel, small talk, or meetings of any kind. I'm an introvert, so they know I need time alone on a daily basis, and that every Mother's Day I skip town and do whatever I want by myself. They also know I love driving my Jeep and listening to music, watching cult documentaries, *Law & Order*, and *Friends*, and they are very clear about my obsession with '80s and '90s pop culture trivia. They may not always agree or join in, but they understand what I love and the joy it brings me.

I'm telling you, girls love seeing their parents laugh and have fun; it brings them so much joy and lets them see their parents in a whole new way. I've watched so many girls relax and release their tension when they see their parents laugh—it touches something deep inside them where the world feels safer, more childlike, and fun. It not only reminds them that we can lead fulfilling lives, but also boosts their confidence in pursuing their own joy when they know we're doing well.

It also helps if our girls see us take pride in our work or approach our lives with a sense of fulfillment. They will also see us feel overwhelmed, annoyed, and sometimes confused—that's to be expected. But it's the core of ourselves that they tap into, our outlook and experience of being in the world.

If we're conveying through our words or actions that life sucks or that we're just trying to get through each day, they won't have much to aspire to—plus, they may feel the need to take care of us. Our jobs don't need to be our ultimate passions, but maybe painting or running is important to us, or volunteering at the school or the local dog shelter is really rewarding. The goal isn't to make everything our absolute favorite, but rather to demonstrate what does hold significance and prioritize and share those aspects in our lives.

As parents, it's important for us to recognize how often we complain to our girls instead of expressing gratitude or appreciation for what we have. We all experience tough days, and often tough years, but we can also discuss how we navigate these challenges and care for ourselves. By emphasizing what we're looking forward to and what brings us happiness, we not only remind our girls that there's much more ahead, but also reassure them of our commitment to our own self-care.

When I was twenty-seven, my dad had an almost deadly heart attack and stroke, and both my sister and I became significant parts of his caregiving until he passed away seventeen years later. Right after he died, my mom was diagnosed with dementia, and we continued to care for her until she passed two years ago. I didn't become a parent until I was thirty-one, so my daughters have only known me as someone who cares for my parents. They've witnessed the tough days, seen me struggle with my own health during the process, and at the same time observed my sense of fulfillment and gratitude for being able to help them.

We've had ongoing discussions about the complexities of these experiences, and mortality, throughout their lives. I don't pretend to be happy all the time, and I don't gloss over the challenges that they have witnessed. What I share is how purposeful and painful aspects of life can coexist, again highlighting the paradox, and that sometimes the hardest things are the most deeply meaningful.

The moments when I've felt most clear and alive have been during crises with my children or parents, knowing that what I'm doing in those moments is all that truly matters. It strips away distractions, making what's most important unmistakably clear. I also live for calm times when there is nothing I have to do and nothing is expected of me, so I can write outside and watch birds all day.

Both experiences are meaningful and will continue to fluctuate throughout life. I understand that my girls may not fully comprehend these significant shifts in life experiences; this kind of awareness develops with age, and their perception of me is just one of many factors shaping their perspectives.

Our girls learn from watching how we live, not from listening to what we say. Prioritizing our own sense of self and joy not only enhances our lives but also inspires them, reminding them that life can remain exciting and that good things are in their future.

CHAPTER 5

Real Stories from My Daughters

When I told my daughters about writing this book, I asked for their input and sought input from their friends. Each of my daughters shared suggestions and stories, and each had at least one issue that deeply affected her and continues to be a learning experience. Feeling inadequate to fully express their personal perspectives, I asked if they would be willing to share their own stories. I wrote a prologue to introduce each of their stories and to reflect on my observations—what I noticed, overlooked, or hoped for—as they unfolded.

In all three of their stories, the most important aspect has been, and continues to be, the ability to discuss what feels hard, sad, or painful. We've had plenty of messy conversations, made mistakes, practiced repairing and apologizing, sought help from others, and even found some humor in the darkness. Real conversations and a willingness to address what's hard can reduce some challenges, though it won't prevent them entirely. Creating a culture of real conversations at home and showing a willingness to engage without judgment can make the most difficult times a little more manageable.

REAL STORIES FROM MY DAUGHTERS

EXPECTATION AND COMPARISON

When Jacey was little and sitting in a high chair in a restaurant, she used to stare at people and observe them for long periods of time. Even when they met her gaze, she wouldn't look away; it was like she was watching them on TV, hidden from view.

She always noticed everything, and it's been fascinating and cool to see how deeply she observes. I can also see how this ability has led to her feeling the pressure of comparison or expectation. She notices what everyone else is doing, she pays attention to what people are saying, and in her generation, there's extreme pressure to excel, with expectations for achievement felt intensely across academics, careers, and personal goals, even without anyone explicitly demanding it.

Jacey and our other two daughters manage their own classes and grades, and Todd and I typically only checked PowerSchool for planning teacher conferences or viewing final report cards. Jacey kept up; she knew how to navigate school. But she lived inside a system that focused on aiming higher, achieving more, striving for the best colleges, or simply staying excessively busy, and she felt the pressure.

She's always had strong gut instincts and could make decisions quickly, but would sometimes second-guess herself after sharing her choices or talking with peers. While it can be beneficial to vet our decisions this way, she often relied too heavily on external opinions, undermining her own intuition. There was often a disconnect between what felt right to her and what society reflected back to her. At her age, it's hard to know what to trust.

COVID hit her high school class hard; they were just getting into their junior year, and they lost so much of their high school experience due to lockdown. She had just started working, really stretching into new experiences, meeting people, exploring opportunities, and then it all came to a halt. She noticed how quiet it became when everything stopped; she could finally hear her thoughts and feel her feelings, and it wasn't always comfortable.

We were all grateful that she was at least able to have an outdoor senior prom and an outdoor graduation ceremony. Knowing that the class before her missed out on many of these rituals and experiences, we felt lucky and appreciative. What her class missed was more time to grow together, and there were breaks in friendships and stifled social development. As things started to open back up, they had to redevelop their skills.

She is now in her senior year, and her major has been a great fit, aligning perfectly with her interests. She's unsure about where it will lead or how it will all unfold, especially now that her friends are pursuing internships and jobs post-college. She can't see how the things she is doing now will connect with a future job, but I like to tell her how my dad would say that life makes more sense in hindsight; things that initially seem insignificant or out of place fit perfectly upon reflection. Our goals and ideas can provide direction, but it's the unplanned experiences we encounter along the way that piece our lives together and make them interesting.

Jacey has been observing those around her confidently discussing their future plans, and she's worried. Her path isn't clear, and she's wondering if she's doing something wrong. As parents, we know that any plans are just that—plans. Life is too unpredictable and ever-changing, and usually, we can never even guess where we will end up.

The one thing we can keep reminding our girls, and what we keep telling Jacey, is to trust themselves, honor when it feels comfortable or uncomfortable, and listen when they feel it's time to step forward or make a change. Jacey knows she needs to take it one step at a time and keep paying attention to herself, but it can be hard to remember when you don't know where it will lead. As Ralph Waldo Emerson said, "To be yourself in a world that is constantly trying to make you something else is the greatest accomplishment."

Jacey's Story

My story centers on the current period of my life, which is both incredible and overwhelmingly challenging. It focuses on the expectation of having a plan during the college years and the amount of comparison we're exposed to from an early age, which is hard to shake off. While this might feel specific to my age, I think anyone can relate to these experiences, regardless of whether they're currently in school or not.

Before I begin, I want to acknowledge my privilege in being able to go to school, have these experiences, and even figure out what I am passionate about. I know this is not the case for everybody, and I don't want any of this to sound oblivious.

I graduated high school in 2021. COVID hit in 2020, and that completely stopped everything, obviously, as we know. And in terms of my goals, thoughts, ambitions, ideas of what I wanted to do, all of that kind of stopped, too. I was in the middle of the rat race of being a junior in high school, playing a sport, working a job, doing ACT practice, you know, all the things we are expected to do.

I feel like, before COVID, most people my age were just kind of zooming around and not thinking about what we were doing. It felt less about living and more about getting through. We were kind of going through the motions, and then COVID opened my perspective, like, wow, this is my life, and this has been my life, and everything's just stopped.

During this pause, it really made me rethink the whole eight-hour school day. My friends and I always talk about how crazy high school life is, the expectation is unbelievable. Like, eight-hour days, homework, sports, some sort of extracurricular—in hindsight, it seems ridiculous. And that's the time when we are needing the most sleep because we are growing, which is crazy.

With all of that happening, how am I supposed to know who I am and what I want to do when excessive busyness is my everyday experience? I felt stuck in this cycle of life without a chance to breathe or think. There isn't enough time to discover who I am, yet somehow, I'm expected to know what I want to do with the rest of my life.

It doesn't help that the school system is set up for comparison—it starts really early in elementary school and works its way all the way up into college, into internships, and eventually careers. I had the experience as early as second grade; when the class would go into "reading groups," I would go into another room and get extra reading help. There was a physical and mental separation between my peers and me.

This continued into middle school, where I was placed in higher-level courses, and then in high school, feeling the pressure to strive for honors or AP classes. In a college-prep environment, this was an everyday reality. We constantly compared our every move to others', feeling inadequate unless we were excelling the most.

Not to mention having a phone attached to our hip throughout this whole process. There is too much to say about social media, but I will say this: it's like having another job. There goes a significant percentage of your emotional, physical, mental, spiritual well-being watching everyone be "happier" than you are and becoming more "successful" than you are every single day. I know it's an illusion, but it still affects us.

My first day of high school was a half-day, and I walked into the auditorium feeling super nervous. I, along with the rest of my freshman class, listened as seniors and staff talked to us about preparing for college. First day, fourteen years old, and they are already telling me to prepare for college.

And I thought to myself, *that's insane, I just got here. Like, that's really what we're going to be talking about on the first day of our freshman year?* I just realized how we're never able to live in the present moment and think for ourselves right here, right now. We're constantly trained to think about two or three years in the future, and it continues to affect and sidetrack me, especially at this point in my life.

I was fortunate to know exactly where I wanted to go to college, so I applied to one school, got accepted, and was excited to attend. It wasn't a difficult decision, for which I'm incredibly grateful. And I thought, perfect, here we go.

I also entered college undecided, which I'm really proud of. When you go in undecided, you can figure things out as you take classes, and that's a big gift you can give yourself, especially at eighteen, when you might not know all the options. Up to that point, I felt like I had been following others and doing what others told me to do, without considering what I truly wanted to do, so taking my time with a major felt right.

I do admire young people who go into school knowing what they want to do; I think it's amazing. I just can't relate, which is why I went in without declaring anything. After taking some classes and exploring possible majors during my freshman year, I discovered a major that sounded interesting. Everything I loved seemed to fit under global studies and social impact. Interestingly, not many people at my university even know this major exists. I was fortunate to have parents who told me that you're going to school to figure out what you want to do, not just to prepare for a career, so just follow what pulls you.

So that's what I did. I decided to go for it, and I didn't really think much of it. Then sophomore year comes along, and I did so much that year, I was so busy. I had classes, a job, a sorority, important relationships to maintain—it was a lot, and it was kind of a blur.

Then, junior year, I knew I was going to study abroad. I'd known I wanted to study abroad since I was like sixteen, probably earlier, for real. That was my number one goal, the thing I knew I wanted to do. I wanted to go to Italy, live with an Italian family, speak Italian, and travel all over Europe. I wanted to immerse myself in another place and get uncomfortable and try every new thing I could.

It's the thing I knew for sure, and it was the only thing I thought about. I finally go, and it was one of the hardest things I've ever done, but also the most rewarding thing I've ever done. It was a goal that I personally planned, worked for, and accomplished. For so many reasons, it's a time that I will cherish for the rest of my life.

But now I am post-abroad, getting ready to start my senior year in college. After I got back, that's when life slowly crept back to me and I was like, wow, I graduate in a year. That's terrifying. Maybe I regret my major. I regret all the money I've spent on this. I don't know what I'm doing. I'm getting questions from people who say things like, *What's your major? Ooh, what are you going to do with that? Never really heard of that...how are you going to use it?*

I don't know. Should I know? It planted so much doubt in me this past semester. My family and close friends understand why I love my major, but the outside world, people who didn't really know me, other adults that

REAL STORIES FROM MY DAUGHTERS

I may talk to, they are so intent on questioning, which is super frustrating because I'm actually going to school for something I am passionate about. I just don't know how to answer their questions, I don't know yet.

And that freaked me out. I was like, this is, this is not good. I need to rethink what I've done.

A lot of my friends and people around me have chosen pre-professional majors with clear next steps—teaching, nursing, advertising, physical therapy, accounting. They've paved a different path than mine, which has also caused a lot of doubt for me. I'm like, wow, the people around me know exactly what they're going to do, and here I am still figuring things out. I question if the things they're pursuing are what they are really passionate about, or maybe I'm projecting because I don't know my own next step.

With all that said, a parent's support—or lack thereof—can profoundly shape our mentality, for better or worse. Many parents advise their kids to enjoy this phase of life, but it can actually be quite stressful. People often reminisce about this time, college, twenties, as fun, forgetting that we're uncertain about what lies ahead. We lack the life experience to fully grasp how to navigate what's coming and whether it will turn out okay.

Also, yes, yes, you were our age once, but you didn't grow up in the time we are living in now. So please don't compare. I think the glamorization of our twenties by adults and the media is hard because it makes us feel like we're doing something wrong if we're not happy all the time. That's frustrating, because there are obviously amazing times, incredible experiences, self-exploration, realizations, and a life where my friends are like my family, but it's not all happy and shiny. We struggle, too. I wish we could struggle without people telling us we should be happy. That just makes the struggle feel bigger.

It helps when I remember that I am going to do this with my friends, that it is going to be okay. I'm doing this with a team; we're not doing this alone. And we hope that our parents will be on our team, too, that they understand that this time is hard. Although everything seems like it's at the tip of our fingers and we have all the opportunity in front of us, it can feel like a lot, almost too many choices. It's hard to know if we are doing it right.

Parents who are asking all those unknowable questions—*where are you going to live, what job are you going to pursue, how will you make money, what are your goals, what's next*—seem to be putting their own worries on their kid. I've seen how this can be detrimental; I watch my friends really struggle when their parents pressure them. This is a time when we really need support, to be told we can do it, that we have skills, and we have what it takes to figure it out. It's such a vulnerable time and having people who believe in us makes a big difference, it reminds us we are capable.

It's a place we've never been before, being on our own and having to choose things for ourselves. When the people who are supposed to support us end up being the ones to tear us down, express more fear than us, or become excessively demanding, it becomes doubly challenging. It adds another weight to worry about, another issue to manage.

I know that many parents fear their child is failing because they've consciously or unconsciously built up these expectations in their minds. When expectations aren't met, parents start to worry. If their kids don't have a complete plan, or if it doesn't look the way the parents expected, the parents can't deal with their own anxiety, leaving the kids to manage their lives and their parents' feelings about their lives. It's so hard to carry other people's emotions; it's hard enough to carry our own.

I think if I could tell the parents out there anything, it would be to give your kids some space and grace to grow into themselves. Let it be difficult for them and support them when they need it. I'm not just talking about money support; I'm talking about love and trust. I also know that college is not for everybody, there are many paths, many ways to figure out who we are and what we love. I hope parents can be open to that, too.

I've learned from the people around me—my parents, my friends, my professors—that success isn't linear, and opportunities are all around us. They say to keep a lookout because opportunities will present themselves when the time is right. I believe them, but I can't see it yet; I don't know how it works because I'm not there.

I think the most important things I've learned about myself aren't related to my career, goals, or future. Instead, I've gained insights into my emotional well-being, managing my anxiety, choosing the right people to surround myself with, discovering what truly benefits me, and finding the schedule that suits me best. All of these aspects of personal contentment aren't really things people teach you directly, you just naturally figure them out along the way. That's where I wish I could focus more of my attention, rather than on more career goals and another five-year plan.

I feel like these important, everyday things, these emotional aspects of our lives, get cast aside, especially during these early adult years, when in my opinion, emotions are at their highest. I wish we had more space to not know, to be able to fail without paralyzing fear. We need to hear that it's okay that we don't know, or that we aren't sure. I trust I am going to figure it out, we all will, but all I can handle right now is my next step.

APPEARANCE

When Camryn was in fourth grade, she had to wear a bulky and uncomfortable expander to start the process of orthodontic work. It was painful and difficult for her to talk, and it was a constant adjustment and definitely inconvenient when it came to eating. Over the years she had more dental and orthodontic work than her sisters combined, and we admired how hard she worked to adapt to it all.

One day that year, while already coping with her mouth expander, she had a reaction to something that resulted in a rash on her face. The rash was red, uncomfortable, and itchy, adding yet another layer of discomfort to her feelings and appearance.

Despite everything, she woke up for school, had breakfast, and was ready to leave on time. When she hopped out of the car, her friends greeted her, and they all walked into school chatting and laughing. After school, she came home and did her homework, had dinner, and went to bed. She had very few complaints, but we also knew it was a tough day. She persevered with remarkable resilience, which was typical of her.

Back in elementary school, Camryn wore whatever she wanted, and there was this yellow sweater she absolutely loved. She's nineteen now and it of course doesn't fit her anymore, but she still keeps it in her closet at home. That sweater reminds her of a time when she didn't care so much, when things didn't get to her. Kids used to tease her about wearing it all the time, but that just made her wear it even more. She didn't really care what anyone thought back then; she had her own way of seeing things.

At fifteen, when her skin started breaking out, she was concerned, but I normalized her experience in my own mind. My own skin had broken out when I was a teen, her peers' skin was breaking out—it all seemed quite typical. I remember my own days of buying Clearasil, Noxzema, and Stridex pads; it was a rite of passage to figure out how to manage your skin.

REAL STORIES FROM MY DAUGHTERS

We supported her trying new over-the-counter medicines, but over time, she felt her skin was getting much worse, and I was getting worried about her stamina. I could see she was losing faith, trying everything, and blaming herself. It was her junior year, with so much already on her plate. She would share how her skin made her confidence plummet, leaving her exhausted by the end of every day.

Her resilience wasn't lacking; the situation was just too overwhelming. She needed support to be seen and understood. Asking her to be indifferent to her appearance only made her feel worse. She told me that reassuring her that her experience was normal, or that I hadn't really noticed her skin, wasn't helpful at all. It left her feeling isolated, needing us to understand the emotional toll her skin was taking on her mental well-being.

We first took some steps with a dermatologist that were noninvasive and topical, and when those didn't work, they recommended starting Accutane. Let's just say that Accutane is a commitment. It involves monthly blood tests, daily pills, and side effects like back pain, fatigue, and extremely dry skin and lips. Camryn had most of the side effects, but she was committed.

We watched her navigate everything with remarkable dignity. She would get frustrated by the process, but despite facing constant discouragement, she kept going. Like when she realized the importance of taking Accutane with food for maximum effectiveness—something she hadn't been doing—she felt deflated, fearing she had wasted time or diminished her chances of clearing up her skin. But she eventually integrated what she needed to do and moved forward.

Eventually, her skin began to clear in a way that allowed her to feel like herself again. She didn't need perfect skin; she just needed some sense of control, to know that it could improve and that things could at least get better, maybe a little easier, over time.

I think she sees this time as pivotal in many ways, and it was equally transformative for us. It's reassuring to witness our daughters' strength and resilience, but it's equally important to notice when they can no longer bear the burden alone and need our understanding and support. One of the hardest things is for them to feel like they're carrying everything alone, with no one who understands or who is willing to help them find a way forward. It's also tough when your past resilience makes others overlook your current need for support.

This isn't just a struggle for teenagers—people of all ages are affected by changes in appearance. What seems ordinary to one person can be deeply distressing for another. It's not just about our own thoughts on the subject or how we think we would manage it; it's about listening to what someone is telling us, believing them, and then staying close to them and helping any way we can.

Camryn's Story

Acne held me back from feeling confident in my skin when I was a teen. It started during COVID, when my clear skin suddenly broke out. At first, I thought it would clear up on its own, no big deal, but over time, it just kept getting worse. I tried every acne product, scrub, and skincare routine out there, but nothing seemed to help.

I finally told my parents how much it was bothering me, and we eventually went to the dermatologist. I was given so many different topical treatments and antibiotics, but none of them really worked. My skin would clear up a bit at first, but then it would just purge again, leaving it dry and red. It was super frustrating and made me feel so defeated every time a new treatment didn't work.

I struggled with confidence when I looked in the mirror. I couldn't accept that people saw me that way every day. I worried that others would see me as ugly or think I didn't take care of my skin, but I was doing everything I could to take care of it. It might seem like an exaggerated reaction or excessive focus on my face, but I couldn't ignore the fact that it defined how I looked every day.

For years, I made sure photos of me were only taken from far away, and I avoided mirrors as much as I could. When I did look in the mirror, I always dimmed the lighting to the lowest setting to hide my acne from myself.

I lost count of how many times I put on makeup in such dim light that I couldn't even see which products I was using. It was all to avoid really looking at my face. Sometimes, I'd try to check for progress or look out of curiosity, but those moments usually ended with me in tears and then retreating to my room. If I had a day when I felt terrible about my face, I wouldn't want to go to school, go to the mall, or do anything that involved leaving the house. All I wanted to do was hide from everybody.

My biggest pet peeve during that time was when I told someone about my skin struggles, and they would mention that they never even washed their face and still had perfect skin. It was another reminder that it must be my fault, something I was doing wrong. Or when my mom would say it's not that bad, or that she doesn't really notice it when she looks at me. I knew it wasn't the first thing she thought about when she looked at me, but I knew it was there, and I needed her to know how much it affected me.

There was a time when I went to summer camp for two weeks, which is one of my favorite things to do each year. It was during a period when my skin was at its worst. I hoped those two weeks away would help me relax and escape from all the anger and frustration I felt because at camp, nobody really cares how they look.

It's upsetting to me that two years later, I can't recall a single story or experience from those two weeks that isn't filled with shame and disappointment about my appearance. I started to shrink my life because of how deeply sad I felt.

I knew that there were very few things we could control in this world, but I was under the impression that I could at least control what I say, what I do, and how I present myself. The fact that I had absolutely no control over how my skin looked was mind-boggling and really devastating to me. It didn't make sense that I could be doing all the right things and still be failing.

Eventually, I started Accutane, which is quite a serious drug and considered a last resort. It has plenty of side effects, and I had to undergo monthly blood tests while on it. I was willing to take it because I was so tired of cycling through shame, sadness, hopefulness, and still feeling crushed.

Throughout the roughly two years of my skin journey, I believed that once I had perfect skin, I would be happy, and confident, and everything would be better. Of course, this turned out to be mostly BS because once that aspect of my life was resolved, I somehow ended up finding other things to feel insecure about.

It's easier to go out feeling confident now, but clearing up my acne didn't magically fix everything like I thought it would at fifteen. Those same insecure feelings now come up in other parts of my life—things I never even worried about when I had acne. Insecurities seem to like finding new places to settle.

I don't know why I felt so worthless just because I couldn't live up to the perfect standard I thought I was supposed to meet. Maybe it was about trying to control who I was, especially during lockdown when everything else was out of control.

Now, when I look in the mirror with the lights on, I do my best to cut myself some slack. I spent so much time tearing down my fifteen-year-old self for something that wasn't my fault. I'm not kinder to myself just because my acne is gone. I try to be kinder because I've figured out that getting mad at yourself for something you can't change only messes with your head and makes you lose track of who you really are.

EATING

When my youngest daughter was in seventh grade, she told me that she had an eating problem. She explained that she was having difficulty eating things she wanted and that she had gone through periods of time without eating anything at all. I was called into the school counselor's office because that's where she first shared what she was going through.

I told her that I had noticed some things, but I still didn't really understand. I reflected on the previous night when she seemed to have eaten plenty, and in doing so, I failed to grasp the significance of the moment and what she was telling me. When we drove home from the school, I asked her in passing if she wanted to go to Starbucks and grab something to eat.

She looked at me like I was crazy, like, *Don't you understand what I just said?* After many more difficult conversations where she went into detail about her feelings and struggles, I realized my daughter was telling me she had an eating disorder. This felt unreal for many reasons, but mostly because, well, I'm a therapist and I would have noticed if she had an eating disorder. I work with women with have had eating disorders, and I talk to young girls about eating and body image. I'm with my daughter every day, and we talk all the time. I know her well.

For a time, I just kept calling it disordered eating because this couldn't be an eating disorder. But it was, and it took me a while to fully grasp it. I had noticed that she picked at her food, ate sometimes far away from us or at odd times, but I kept chalking it up to adolescent behavior or picky eating. I did see it, but I didn't know what I was looking at, or refused to consider what I was seeing. I had no idea that she had started investigating calories on her phone, that she had a bag of candy in her closet that she wanted so badly to eat but felt like she couldn't, and that her Instagram algorithm was sending her ways to eat less, work her body, and avoid any kind of food that wasn't "clean" or "healthy."

This meant that not only did my daughter need help, but I did too. It was confusing because we prided ourselves on avoiding discussions about diets, weight obsession, and appearance, which were common in my generation. Todd and I have lived together for over twenty years without ever owning a scale. But there's more to eating disorders than what we say at home. I had to move beyond preconceived ideas about why eating disorders take hold (it's not always about appearance), what they actually look like (it's not always obvious), and how they affect and alter the brain.

While my clinical training had taught me that eating disorders were connected to anxiety, I had to learn about how they shift the way we process the world and how they lead to intense isolation, shame, and create a cycle of denial and pain. I didn't realize that many general practitioners don't recognize the signs of eating disorders and can inadvertently add stress by immediately weighing kids, assessing their BMI, praising them for being a certain weight, or expressing concern if they aren't, all within the first five minutes of an appointment.

I also didn't know that most therapists, including myself, haven't been properly trained to understand, treat, or talk about eating disorders, and often end up not being as knowledgeable or supportive of clients as we should be.

Eating disorders are among the deadliest mental illnesses and can be very difficult to treat, often depending on how long mindset and behaviors have been present. Research has shown that the pandemic worsened eating disorders and heightened levels of anxiety and depression.

On the bright side, I also learned, and personally witnessed, that full recovery is completely possible, something that most people assume isn't true. The misconception that quitting drinking, drugs, or other addictions is easier than addressing eating disorders comes from the mistaken belief that merely abstaining from a particular substance resolves the issue. But it's not that simple.

Yes, someone can stop drinking, but the real challenges of alcoholism and addiction lie in the mental, social, and physical dependencies that come with it. Similarly, with eating disorders, it's not just about eating. These disorders are like a tangled web of emotions, body image issues, and self-esteem struggles. Fixing it requires more than just changing food habits. It involves digging into the psychological roots and finding new coping mechanisms. Becoming educated as a therapist, and parent, was the beginning of a more profound understanding of how an eating disorder stems from a combination of genetic, biological, psychological, and environmental factors.

It was also the beginning of our relationship with other families and experts in the eating disorder community, and most importantly, a therapist and dietitian who specialized in eating disorders and guided my daughter and our family every step of the way. We have been swimming in the world of diet culture our whole lives, so uncovering the true meaning of normal eating was a heavy lift, and having experts who have seen the same things over and over and know what works long-term provided a sense of grounding and sanity.

There is a difference between eating disorders and disordered eating. Think of it as a continuum with intuitive eating on one side, where someone eats to fuel themselves and have a completely balanced relationship with food, and way on the other end of the continuum you've got diagnosed eating disorders. In the middle lies disordered eating, which includes behaviors and beliefs around food that cause issues but may not be reaching the level of a full-blown disorder.

All these behaviors are normalized on social media, which specifically targets young girls to follow accounts promoting eating, exercise, and weight loss. Social media did play a role in Skylar's eating disorder; she had just started using it earlier that year. During her treatment, she decided to take several years away from social media and has only recently resumed minimal engagement.

Both eating disorders and disordered eating are used as an escape from life's pain and discomfort. It becomes a means to fixate on what we perceive as controllable when everything else feels chaotic. Society's fixation on the ideal of "optimal" performance exacerbates this issue, and we're conditioned to believe that we only deserve food if we meet certain standards, rather than recognizing that eating encompasses more than mere survival—it's about experiencing joy, connection, and overall well-being.

Our home was full of learning and change, and we knew we had to share it with the people we loved most so they could be part of it with us. "No secrets" became our motto, allowing us to openly discuss eating and allowing my daughter to share her feelings every step of the way. Every three months or so, we'd send an email to our loved ones, keeping them updated on progress and what we were learning. This helped our family stay informed and made it easier to talk about my daughter's experience during family gatherings, reducing any awkwardness or discomfort.

While Skylar's anorexic behaviors were being deconstructed over a relatively short period of time, mostly because she had only been practicing restrictive behaviors for only four months before she told us, she still deals with ARFID, which stands for avoidant/restrictive food intake disorder (ARFID), which means she is more selective based on sensory avoidance with food tastes, textures, temperature and smells. With hindsight, we see that she was struggling with ARFID in early childhood, but it was too easy to qualify it as picky eating and as something normal for a young child.

My daughter has incorporated what she's learned about anxiety and its connection to eating into her daily life. She's good at noticing and talking about her feelings, and she's good at recognizing when she needs new coping skills or some kind of support from adults. As a family, we've gained a deeper understanding of how prevalent diet culture is. We've noticed how even well-intentioned people promote restrictive eating habits like cleanses, fasts, clean eating, and paleo diets, making it nearly impossible for young people, or old people, to avoid feeling guilty about their food choices or appearance. It's important to point out that eating disorders aren't exclusively a concern for girls—eating disorders have surged among boys, nearly reaching the same level as girls.

As a podcaster and writer, my daughter's journey was not for public consumption, so, while we were open with family and close friends, we didn't share on social media or on our show. It was her story, and it still is. She said she wanted to share this story in the book because now, almost five years later, she believes that sharing could benefit young girls struggling with the same things she did and give parents insight into how to understand or support their kids more effectively.

No single way of eating is right because every body has unique needs, just as there's no correct appearance because bodies are naturally diverse in size and shape. I know these sentiments sound cliché, everybody says it, but not enough of us believe it or live it. I've noticed that those who truly get this concept are people who have faced serious diagnoses, battled long-term illnesses, or are aging and experiencing declines in physical health. Their profound appreciation and understanding of their bodies goes beyond societal norms; they prioritize function and gratitude above all else.

As a family, our experience of figuring out what "normal eating" means aligns very well with all the messages in this book. There isn't one correct path, definitive answer, or universally shared experience when it comes to feeding ourselves. We do our best to focus on listening to our bodies and understanding their needs, typically known as intuitive eating, rather than blindly following trends or diets promoted by influencers who don't know anything about us.

The big-picture goal is to adopt an approach to eating that prioritizes moment-to-moment well-being. This can help us decrease our thinking about food and eating to a more proportional size, and not allow it to take up so much space in our brains and lives. At the start of our journey, our daughter's dietitian shared this essay by Ellyn Satter as a daily reminder of how to engage with eating—it's still prominently displayed on our refrigerator.

> Normal eating is going to the table hungry and eating until you are satisfied. It is being able to choose food you like and eat it and truly get enough of it—not just stop eating because you think you should.

Normal eating is being able to give some thought to your food selection, so you get nutritious food, but not being so wary and restrictive that you miss out on enjoyable food. Normal eating is giving yourself permission to eat sometimes because you are happy, sad or bored, or just because it feels good.

Normal eating is mostly three meals a day, or four or five, or it can be choosing to munch along the way. It is leaving some cookies on the plate because you know you can have some again tomorrow, or it is eating more now because they taste so wonderful. Normal eating is overeating at times, feeling stuffed and uncomfortable. And it can be undereating at times and wishing you had more. Normal eating is trusting your body to make up for your mistakes in eating.

Normal eating takes up some of your time and attention but keeps its place as only one important area of your life. In short, normal eating is flexible. It varies in response to your hunger, your schedule, your proximity to food and your feelings.

The handout, "What is Normal Eating?" is © 2018 by Ellyn Satter. Published at www.Ellynsatterinstitute.org. The Ellyn Satter Institute is the official source for the interpretation and application of the Satter feeding and eating models. For additional information, please visit ellynsatterinstitute.org.

Skylar's Story

I don't really know how to start, but I guess I'll start with my experience and how the eating disorder started. I think it's different for everybody; this is just my story. What I've learned from therapy is that whenever people's eating disorders start, it's usually not about body image.

It's more like something bad is happening in your life at the time and then you latch on to whatever you can to stay afloat, and for me during COVID, I latched on to an eating disorder. During COVID I felt lonely, and I felt like I didn't have anything I was doing right. For some reason I decided that my stomach didn't look good enough, it actually looked like it was getting bigger, so maybe I could just latch on to fixing that.

It started for me in early fall, and it was kind of healthy at first, like I was just trying to be healthier and have something to focus on. So I started doing these workouts and it felt pretty normal, and then it started to change.

I was trying my best to do everything correctly, to be healthy in every way. To notice some kind of difference in my stomach. But when you're in your eating disorder state of mind, your stomach will never look good enough.

So at that point I decided to try and actually lose weight, and there were so many different diets and things on social media. I had just gotten social media that year when I turned thirteen, and my algorithm had new ideas every day. I tried a lot of different things, and I eventually got to a place where I decided maybe I wouldn't eat at all.

I literally made a decision to not eat. The weird thing is that I knew a fair amount about eating disorders, and I kind of knew this might be a sign of an eating disorder, but I still felt like it was something I should do, so I could reach my goal quickly.

I felt bad right away and I started feeling like I was going to faint. Then I started counting all my calories and doing even more intensive workouts. I didn't even think I was doing that much at the time because I never felt like I was doing the eating disorder good enough. I felt like I was failing in some way. I was self-aware enough to know that this probably had to end at some point, I just didn't know when. Then I started getting really skinny and I noticed my ribs were starting to show, and I felt like that's when I started to gauge where my eating disorder was at, based on how much of my rib cage I could see.

That's when I felt like I was actually doing it correctly, when it physically showed, and I could actually see it in my body. Then I started feeling good, like, *I'm doing this correctly, it's actually working*, and it felt like something good I could focus on during this time. I was really fuzzy—I don't even remember that much of it because you can't process memory if you're hungry all the time, but there was a type of fulfillment that I experienced. But again, it was COVID, and I was so bored and had nothing to do during the day. Luckily, I had a friend to Facetime and talk to like all the time, which was really great, but there was just nothing to do during COVID, so I would just sit in my room.

That's where I feel like I am different from other people with eating disorders. Others had to hide from their friends, and because it was COVID and I didn't have to go out, I didn't have to hide it. I barely had to hide it from my family. I didn't feel good about myself, and then there were days where I was worried about dying in my sleep. I was worried that I just would stop breathing because of my lack of eating, and I didn't really want to die. I just wanted to feel like I was actually doing this well. Then our family friend had to go to the hospital for an eating disorder, and that kind of broke me. I felt like she was doing it better than me, like, she actually needs to get help, so I must not be doing this correctly.

I was doing all kinds of workouts; I was running steps, and I was working out while watching TV. Nothing was ever good enough, and I wanted to stop. I didn't really want to eat, but then it felt weird to not want to eat, because I wanted to grow and get healthy.

I was just hungry, and I did know that this would have to end at some point. I knew enough about eating disorders that this wasn't good, and I think I needed some attention because I had been doing this for several months.

I made a few different plans to get help, writing letters to my parents and a few friends, but I settled on telling my school counselor. I wrote her a letter. I don't even know where that letter is, but I gave it to her, and she read it in front of me. I was like, *oh my god, my entire world just crashed.* I just admitted to every single thing that has been keeping me going. Then my mom came to the school and the first thing that she said was, *I know.*

I thought I was being so good at it because when everyone was having dinner, I'd have an apple, so I was like yeah, they probably noticed something. I didn't like when my parents told me they knew more about my eating disorder than I did, or that I was not alone. They took me to the hospital, and I had to get lots of tests to make sure I was physically healthy. I had to get my heart checked and I had to get my blood drawn and that was a really tough day because I was just like, my entire everything is just done, and this is the thing that's been keeping me going for months. It's just over, and that night was awful because I was just in so much pain and I was still so hungry. I hadn't eaten all day and I had to like sip this chocolate thing that my mom got me, and I just hated it.

I was like, this is awful, and then the next morning my mom took me to the chiropractor, and she said to me "I know you're still in there" because I was a shell of myself, and I remember it so distinctly. I don't even remember how I felt about that because I thought I was who I was because of the eating disorder, so it was confusing.

I think the first thing that had made me even slightly happy was one day my sister came into my room and asked me if I wanted any of her bread. I was just so happy that she had asked me, and it tasted really good. All day my parents had shown that they cared about me, and they assured me they were going to take care of me, but my sister offering me some of her food was sweet, because she didn't know how else to help me. She made me feel like I was an important person, and that was the first time I had felt even a little bit happy in like four months.

Then my mom and I went on a walk, and I realized I felt guilty about eating that bread. But I was still like, okay, we're just going to have to do whatever we need to get through this. I was only in seventh grade, and I didn't really know what was going to happen next, but we started figuring it out as we went.

The first couple days we didn't really know what the plan was, we didn't know what we were going to do. We considered the hospital, but the program was for teens and adults, and I had never really done therapy. My mom learned about family-based treatment (FBT), where you eat at home and your family makes sure you eat and stick to a plan. At first, I was given very like small amounts of food. Like I remember being given one egg at breakfast.

We didn't really know what to do, so we were just trying our best to figure this out. My parents would play Uno with me all day, we'd go on walks, and we'd journal about what was good about the day. I was just trying my best to get by. I was quiet a lot of the time and I had a lot of mood swings.

Then we went to a therapist who wasn't so great, because she wasn't trained in how to help with eating disorders, and it was obvious. In a week, I actually felt like I was recovered because I was eating. But I still didn't want to eat, but my parents were feeding me what I now remember as really small amounts just so I would eat something.

The one thing I didn't like was that my mom kept calling it disordered eating, and it took her awhile to call it an eating disorder. I was so mad because part of the reason this even happened was because I wanted to be good at something, and if I didn't even have an eating disorder, then maybe I just made all of this up?

I know this isn't everybody's experience, but that was mine. I just didn't like being told about my own experience. So many therapists were booked up, but about three weeks into my recovery, we finally found a therapist and a dietitian who were trained in eating disorders, and I still work with them today.

Initially I would see them weekly, and my dietitian gave my parents and me a clear plan of what I was supposed to be eating. It was a lot more than what I had been eating for the last couple of weeks. The idea was that food is medicine, and initially I had to eat a lot more than your average person eats just to get my body back on track. I had to refuel because a brain doesn't think right when it's been starved. It literally cannot think, and that's why I don't remember a lot of details from this time.

My dietitian would have me track what I was eating, and she gave us a clear idea of what to eat. We came up with a bunch of meal plans. I don't even remember what my therapist and I started talking about at the beginning, but it was focused on trying to get to the bottom of why this occurred and what are we going to do about it now.

I missed a couple of weeks of school, and at home we just followed a plan and focused on eating. Every night my mom and I would make a plan for the day—for literally every single moment of the day—so there was no moment when I didn't know what we were going to do next.

Every day we would figure out exactly what I would eat and when. We did this for a long time. After about four months, my dietitian told me to stop planning what I was going to eat and start practicing real-life eating. I was gaining weight and getting better, and by then I was okay with gaining weight—not because I liked it, but I was like, well, I'm not the one doing this, it's other people telling me what to do, so I can't blame myself.

Everyone was looking out for me, and I was only going to school part-time. My school counselor was really helpful and understanding. Sometimes it would be one step forward and a few steps back, and that's okay. I knew that I should recover, but even while I was recovering, I was finding ways to hold the eating disorder, like I would sneak out to work out in the basement, or I would still count my calories. I still had all these control issues, even as I was recovering.

The first thing that made me think that I really needed to get better was when my dietitian told me that my cousin Claire, who was super helpful during the time, wouldn't like me better if I had an eating disorder. This wasn't a thing to scare me, she just said, if you don't go up to get food at Thanksgiving, Claire is not going to think you're a cooler or better person because you're not going up to get food. That felt insane to me, because I thought I would be a better person if I didn't eat as much. But realizing that Claire wouldn't think this was cool kind of blew my mind. I was like, oh, I actually have to get fully better, not just a little better.

At the beginning, everyone had to watch me eat, make sure I ate, and now I'm just normally eating, and it's been that way for almost five years. It took a while to figure everything out, and sometimes I still think about it, but I don't count calories anymore and I don't notice calories on the menu.

It's not really about food anymore, I can go a long time without thinking about my body image or what I'm eating. I do see that a lot of people I know have eating disorders—up until last year it was really triggering to me, but now I feel more sad for them. I know I don't have the power to fix them myself, but I do draw attention to it occasionally, like point out what they say or correct them. But I can't really fix it for them, so I just have to let it be.

Body image is a big deal right now because people think, and I'm not immune to this, that your worth is based on how attractive you are—that a lot of it is based on your body and your face and how you look. I'm strong enough at this point that it doesn't affect me nearly as much as it used to, but it's still a thing I have to get through. It's a very high school thing. But I still believe that it's just going to continue getting better.

It's not that I'm glad that this happened, because there are things I still struggle with that have nothing to do with eating. Eating was just what I was clinging to at the time, the thing I could control and that would help me get by. That's what I did, so I guess it made me who I am. But I also hate it when people say that it made me who I am, because I'm like, it was an eating disorder—I don't care that it made me who I am, because it sucked to get into it, and it sucked to get out of it—so I don't like when people tell me to be glad that it happened, because I'm not really glad it happened.

But the eating disorder helped me in some good ways. I've connected with people who still mean a lot to me. Sometimes I will have days that I completely forget that this was even an issue. In some ways I am happy that my family and I went through this together, it made me feel closer to them.

I'm also just so glad that I don't have to deal with it anymore. I deal with other things, like I still have anxiety and I still have things that I feel like I need to control. I still feel like I have to prove myself in order to be good at something. But I've learned from my therapists that this is very human and doesn't really go away, so they help me work through the feelings.

I'm glad that I had my family with me, and we got closer. I'm glad that I can do things now that I couldn't do before, and I think part of the reason for my happiness is being able to compare how much better I'm doing and how far I've come. But I'm never like, "Yay! I had an eating disorder!" It's not a fun, good thing. The only good thing was my parents, my sisters, my therapists, and the rest of my family helping me get back.

CONCLUSION

Prioritize the Relationship

~~~~~~

Author and spiritual teacher Richard Rohr's concept of the *order, disorder, reorder* wisdom pattern offers a framework for understanding the communication process. We enjoy and appreciate order, and rely on familiar ways of connecting, but as our girls grow, and face various social and societal pressures, there will be inevitable times of disorder, when their needs and perspectives are evolving. During these times, we need to practice adapting with openness, patience, and curiosity, allowing for the discomfort and messiness that comes with disorder.

This paves the way for something new, for a reorder phase where communication deepens, and our relationship evolves accordingly. Embracing this cycle reminds us that navigating these phases is ongoing and integral to meaningful relationships—it's less about whether change will occur and more about how we will handle change when it occurs.

The focus of my work has been bridging the gap between young girls and their parents, guiding them through these cycles of order, disorder, and reorder repeatedly. Too often we normalize unresolved communication breakdowns with teens, digging in our heels about our needs, or just avoiding or pretending the discomfort isn't there. This normalizes and contributes to the chronic defensiveness, anger, or misery that can arise during adolescence. If we fail to pay attention or evolve ourselves during this significant shift, we leave our girls to navigate the learning process on their own.

Without real conversations or repair, unresolved issues can lead to resentment or inherited beliefs that may require therapeutic resolution or may persist indefinitely. Instead, we can explore new ways to communicate and stay connected during this turbulent phase of their lives. Seeking professional support, reading books, and listening to podcasts are beneficial, but it's ultimately our willingness to try new approaches to communication, take initiative, and deepen our understanding that drives meaningful change.

Conflict is inevitable in any significant relationship, and it's particularly true in our relationships with our kids. Our ability to address and resolve these conflicts maturely as our girls grow not only equips them with skills for navigating adult relationships, but it also instills a sense of their own value early on, reassuring them that they matter. This approach prevents them from enduring unnecessary suffering that can lead to harmful cycles later in life—a pattern I frequently observe with my current clients.

Our girls navigate a world not designed with them in mind, and this lack of consideration is reflected in the gender pay gap, gender-based violence, restricted reproductive rights, stereotypes of gender and race inferiority, objectification in media, lack of political representation, and victim-blaming. These factors shift responsibility away from perpetrators and perpetuate harmful attitudes toward women, leaving our girls confused about who they are supposed to be and how they should navigate the world.

PRIORITIZE THE RELATIONSHIP

We can talk with them about their pain and grief, reassuring them that they're not alone and validating that their feelings are completely normal and acceptable. We can promote kindness and community support, reassuring them that their value comes from simply being, not just from what they achieve. We can give them space to talk about their fears and failures without imposing our anxiety on them or invalidating their feelings. That's why the goal of this book is to practice having real discussions, to get ourselves to a place, emotionally and literally, where we can talk about what hurts.

We may have all the wisdom in the world, but if our communication consistently breaks down or if our girls lose respect for us, they become much more unwilling to accept our advice or support. We must be willing to uphold our part of the relationship by acknowledging the energy we bring and our own shortcomings and failures. The more real we are, the more open they will be with us.

In my previous book, *Zen Parenting*, I explored the inevitability of unpredictability. In this book, I emphasize that change is also inevitable. As parents, we can prepare ourselves emotionally, spiritually, and physically to handle these shifts and their ripple effects by trusting in our ability to adapt. While conflict and change can indeed be uncomfortable, it's surprising how often we underestimate our own resilience and ability to adapt, considering how frequently we've successfully navigated change throughout our lives.

Reflecting on our own lives shows how adaptable we can be, particularly when we consider the unprecedented challenges of COVID-19 and 2020. Despite the unique and often horrendous circumstances, our ability to navigate change remains a testament to our resilience.

My generation, the Gen Xers, often joke about being like "feral children," raised to fend for ourselves in the world. While this made us resilient and self-reliant, we didn't always get the emotional support we needed, and I still see those scars in my adult clients today. Through discussion and treatment, they begin to understand the importance of feeling seen, understood, and appreciated. The goal of treatment is to empower them to find these qualities for themselves and then apply this understanding as they raise their daughters.

Sometimes, when I'm with a client and I emphasize the importance of offering her daughter more compassion or validation, she may share a story about not receiving the attention she needed as a child, and how nobody took the time to listen to her opinions. She might add that despite this, she turned out alright.

But at that moment, she is sitting in my office sharing that she's not alright, and we are working together to address the damage caused by this lack of emotional support. This highlights a common oversight for many parents: thinking that toughening up their children through ongoing hardship is more beneficial than introducing new ways to express love, affirming their children's worth and sense of belonging. Developing a sense of value and belonging doesn't diminish our girls' strength or independence; it helps them develop inner trust and a comfort in their skin so they can take on the world.

In recent years, I've noticed a growing number of estrangements where young people disconnect from their parents because they feel misunderstood or not treated as they deserve. It's a heartbreaking reality, as it's less about a lack of love than an inability to effectively communicate that usually creates this problem.

Establishing communication as a priority lays the foundation for the future. It's an ongoing process, not about getting every conversation "right," but about being willing to engage and committed to staying connected. It's about prioritizing the relationship above all else.

PRIORITIZE THE RELATIONSHIP

One straightforward way to use this book is by asking your girls if they resonate with the "Real Things Girls Want You to Know" chapter. Do they agree with the requests listed in the *Know Me, Support Me, Connect with Me, Trust Me,* and *Laugh with Me* sections? What do they feel is missing from these lists? Simply inviting them to review and confirm or elaborate on these points will initiate an interesting, and hopefully meaningful, conversation.

Instead of girls always asking me, "Will you tell my parents this?" you can now read and learn more about what they are experiencing. You can ask them questions and engage in a new way, with greater awareness and a willingness to navigate conflict and maintain a meaningful relationship. It's a chance to break away from old family patterns and develop a healthy communication style that can be passed on to future generations.

Acknowledgments

~~~

This was the first book I've written since both of my parents passed away, but their optimistic and supportive influence remained strong throughout the process. I am also deeply grateful for the ongoing support from my sister and aunt, who each, in their own unique ways, embody a perfect blend of strength and kindness.

I am thankful to everyone who has listened to the Zen Parenting Radio podcast over the past fourteen years and to those who are part of Team Zen. My work continues to be a beloved job that never feels like work. Discussing what matters most and connecting with like-minded individuals has been an invaluable opportunity and a fortunate way of life.

Working with women and girls over the years has impacted my life through the stories they have shared and the trust they have placed in me. To my college students, many of whom are current or future social workers, I deeply admire how you turn your personal challenges into being a force for good. Being your teacher has been one of my greatest joys.

I am grateful to my agent, Rachel Beck, and to my publisher, Mango, especially Brenda Knight, who has been the greatest pleasure to collaborate with. I am also grateful to Dr. John Duffy, my friend and counterpart as author of *Rescuing Our Sons*, and to Annie Burnside, who

ACKNOWLEDGMENTS

supported me in shaping the tone of this book through our countless coffee talks spanning hours.

To my college girlfriends, who are more like family, you keep me real and laughing. Special thanks to Monisha and Jess for indulging my spontaneous texts, stories, memes, and impassioned discussions about politics, Taylor Swift, and the latest cult documentaries. Your constant engagement and support make my life more enjoyable.

I appreciate and honor all the authors who have written about girls and women, including my friends Rosalind Wiseman and Dr. Shefali. Rachel Simmons opened my eyes when I read *The Curse of the Good Girl* so many years ago, and Mary Pipher remains one of my all-time favorite authors for creating conversations about the unique challenges our adolescent girls face with *Reviving Ophelia*.

To my husband and Zen Parenting partner, Todd, thank you for helping me practice and refine my communication skills and for being the most important person in my life. And to our daughters, Jacey, Camryn, and Skylar, your contributions as writers and your roles as my greatest inspiration shaped the entirety of this book. Please don't ever forget how much you matter.

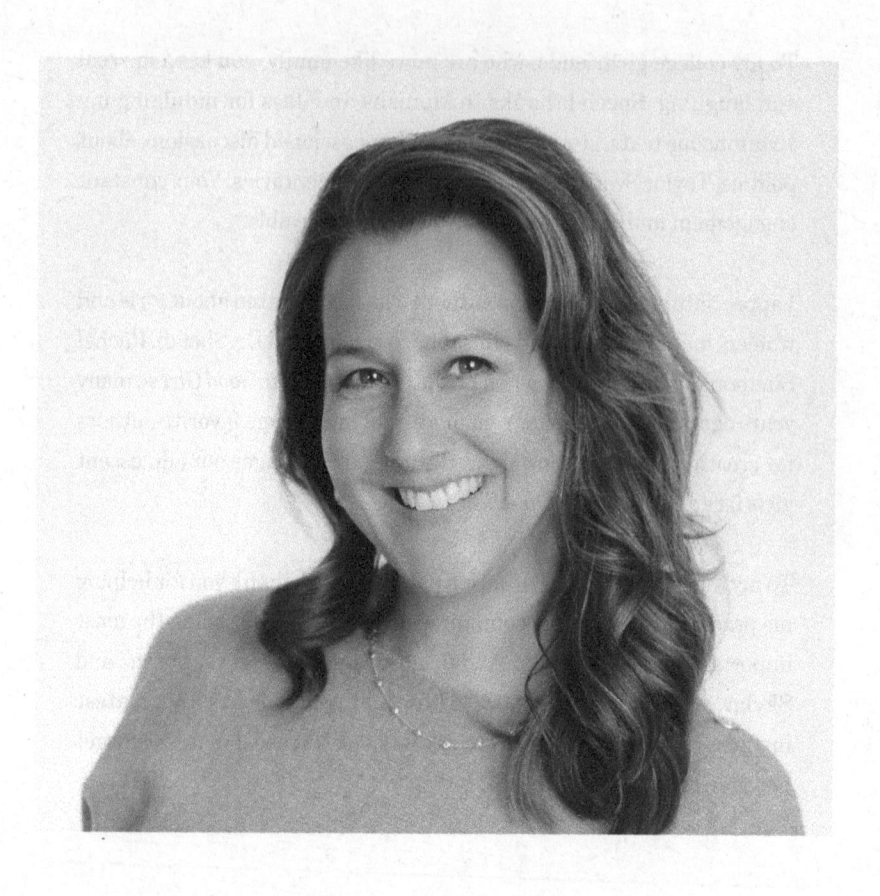

About the Author

~~~~~

Cathy Cassani Adams, LCSW, has cohosted the Zen Parenting Radio podcast, one of the original podcasts about mindful and self-aware parenting, since 2011. She is also the founder of the Zen Parenting Conference in Chicago. Cathy is the author of *Zen Parenting: Caring for Ourselves and Our Children in an Unpredictable World* (2022) and *Living What You Want Your Kids to Learn: The Power of Self-Aware Parenting* (2014), both of which were winners of the Nautilus Award and the International Book Award.

Cathy is a sought-after speaker on parenting and female empowerment, leading women's groups and providing individual support to women and girls. She is a clinical social worker, certified parent coach, former elementary school educator, and yoga teacher. She created and facilitated a self-awareness program for preadolescent girls called Be U and was a child and family therapist and clinical educator at Lurie Children's Hospital of Chicago.

Cathy has been a blogger for the *Huffington Post* and a columnist for *Chicago Parent* magazine, and she currently writes a Substack newsletter called *Zen Parenting Moment*. She was a recurring guest on WGN Radio, and her parent coaching was the focus of a feature article in the *Chicago Tribune* and a CBS News report. She teaches in the Sociology/Criminology Department at Dominican University, and she lives outside of Chicago with her husband Todd and their three daughters.

mango
PUBLISHING

Mango Publishing, established in 2014, publishes an eclectic list of books by diverse authors—both new and established voices—on topics ranging from business, personal growth, women's empowerment, LGBTQ studies, health, and spirituality to history, popular culture, time management, decluttering, lifestyle, mental wellness, aging, and sustainable living. We were named 2019 *and* 2020's #1 fastest growing independent publisher by *Publishers Weekly*. Our success is driven by our main goal, which is to publish high-quality books that will entertain readers as well as make a positive difference in their lives.

Our readers are our most important resource; we value your input, suggestions, and ideas. We'd love to hear from you—after all, we are publishing books for you!

Please stay in touch with us and follow us at:

Facebook: Mango Publishing
Twitter: @MangoPublishing
Instagram: @MangoPublishing
LinkedIn: Mango Publishing
Pinterest: Mango Publishing
Newsletter: mangopublishinggroup.com/newsletter

Join us on Mango's journey to reinvent publishing, one book at a time.

Printed in the USA
CPSIA information can be obtained
at www.ICGtesting.com
JSHW030500151124
73615JS00003B/3

9 781684 816835